THE
EXERCISE
BOOK

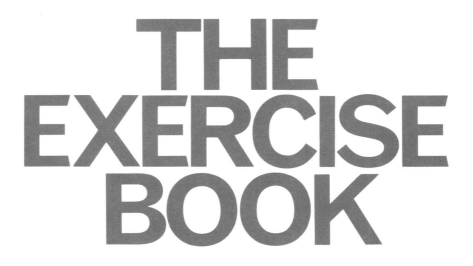

THE EXERCISE BOOK

by Leslie Michener, B.A., B.P.E. and Gerald Donaldson

Photography and design by Peter Christopher

A Jonathan–James Book

Penguin Books

Penguin Books Ltd, Harmondsworth,
Middlesex, England
Penguin Books, 625 Madison Avenue,
New York, New York 10022, U.S.A.
Penguin Books Australia Ltd, Ringwood,
Victoria, Australia
Penguin Books Canada Ltd, 2801 John Street,
Markham, Ontario, Canada L3R 1B4
Penguin Books (N.Z.) Ltd, 182-190 Wairau Road,
Auckland 10, New Zealand

First published by Penguin Books 1978

Copyright © 1978 by Leslie Michener and Gerald Donaldson

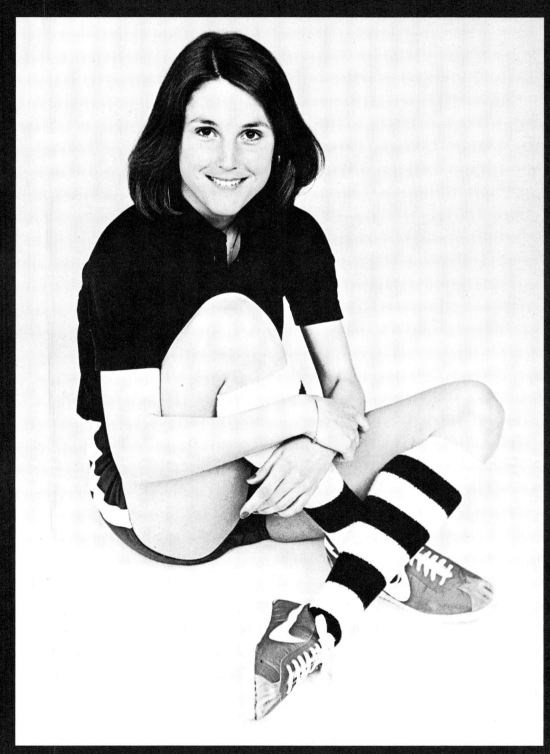

Leslie Michener, B.A., B.P. E.

THE SMILE APPROACH

A smile is a pleasant example of muscular movement. The Exercise Book takes the smile approach to physical fitness.

Your body is designed to move. The Exercise Book moves it with exercises that are logical, natural and as easy as a smile to master. Their flowing and graceful rhythms are satisfying and enjoyable to perform, tension-relieving and smile-provoking — it feels good to move your body this way.

Just as a smile requires less effort than a frown, so does correct movement reduce strain on the body. This is why The Exercise Book avoids jerky movements, never over-stresses any part of your body and relaxes each muscle after involving it in an activity.

The Exercise Book can give you a new awareness of yourself. By acquainting you with the pleasures of being physically fit it can show you that the way you move your body can move your mind. It can improve the way you perceive and the way you're perceived because a body that's fit feels and looks better.

Frowns cause wrinkles. The Exercise Book can remove them and cause smiles all around.

A TECHNICAL EXPLANATION

The Exercise Book is a scientifically devised exercise program to improve the flexibility, strength, endurance, balance, coordination and cardiovascular fitness of men and women of all ages. It consists of forty-eight Movement Patterns, each one involving a sequence of positions that incorporate some combination of strengthening, stretching and/or relaxing different groups of muscles. Four Relaxation Exercises are strategically located within the program.

The program makes use of the inter-relationships of muscular movement: using one muscle group affects another. The coordinated series of exercises involves almost every muscle in the body, sometimes separately and sometimes with several groups of muscles working together.

The muscles of the body are elastic. When they are stretched, they become more flexible which relieves muscular tightness and stress. When contracted, they are strengthened and muscle tone is improved.

The emphasis is on working each muscle group within a comfortable range of activity, relaxing it, then recycling it into another activity. Deep breathing and other forms of relaxing motion enable this to be accomplished with continuous movement, while avoiding fatigue.

The Exercise Book program is one of continuous rhythmical activity. This means that an elevated heart rate can be maintained for cardiovascular fitness. The various elements of each exercise are arranged to avoid excessive repetition, so that stress and boredom are eliminated.

HOW TO USE THE BOOK

1. Learn the exercises: look at the pictures, read the instructions, then practice each sequence. When your instructor is facing you in an exercise involving movement to the right or left, she will make the movement to *your* right or left, so that you can use her as a mirror image.

2. When you have mastered the technique of each exercise, perform them one after the other in the order they appear in the book.

3. Repeat each Movement Pattern from *four* to *twelve* times (depending on your fitness level) unless otherwise noted. Repeat each Relaxation Exercise until you feel recovered and ready to move on.

4. Do the exercises at a comfortable pace, beginning slowly and working harder as you become more fit.

5. Remember not to hold your breath. Usually you should breathe in when expanding your chest, and breathe out when contracting it.

6. Perform each exercise in a smooth, rhythmical fashion, avoiding jerky movements. Concentrate on a fluid transition between each movement.

7. Maintain a reasonable momentum throughout the book. The interval between each exercise should be no longer than it takes you to turn the page.

8. When you have become fit, the complete program in the book should take approximately forty-five minutes to complete.

9. To achieve and maintain a reasonable level of fitness you should do the program from three to five times a week.

10. Always rest if you become unduly fatigued or if you feel strain at any time during the program. Your body will tell you when to stop.

Medical Caution: While The Exercise Book is intended for the use of people of all ages and levels of fitness, it is recommended that you get medical approval if you have been ill, if you are older, or if you have any doubts about your physical condition, before using the book. It's a good idea to have a check-up before engaging in any new form of physical activity. Remember to rest at any time during the exercises if you become unduly fatigued or if you feel strain.

SOME SUGGESTIONS

☐ Before you begin each session with The Exercise Book you should spend a few minutes walking briskly, jogging, cycling or swimming. This loosens up your body, making it more flexible and receptive to the movements in the program, as well as contributing to your overall fitness.

☐ When you finish the program you should relax but keep moving for a few minutes to cool down. A shower or a bath is a good idea hygienically and a pleasant reward for completing your exercise program.

☐ Try to make The Exercise Book a part of your daily routine, fitting it in when convenient so it doesn't become a burden.

☐ A background of music (in 4/4 time) adds enjoyment to the program and contributes to the timing and smooth performance of its rhythmical movements.

☐ A soft surface, such as a mat of foam rubber, is recommended for those exercises which are performed while lying or sitting.

☐ Wear comfortable clothing that allows freedom of movement. Athletic shoes may be worn although they aren't necessary.

1 The first Movement Pattern consists of overhead arm swings with simultaneous knee bends. It strengthens your neck, shoulders and upper back and makes them more flexible. The knee action stretches your calf muscles and thighs while improving your coordination. Develop a 'bouncing' motion in your upper body in B through G by bending your knees as your arms go down and straightening them as your arms come up. Follow the movement of your arm with your eyes.

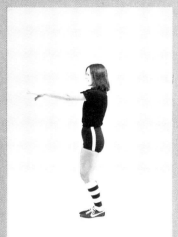

A Stand with your feet together, your knees bent, and your arms forward at shoulder height.

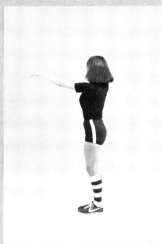

B Raise your right arm in an arc, up, over and behind. Your knees straighten as you raise your arm.

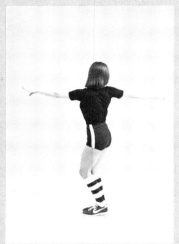

C Finish with your right palm up and your knees bent again.

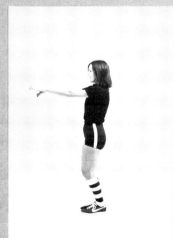

D Return to **A** by swinging your arm back the way it came, straightening and then bending your knees again.

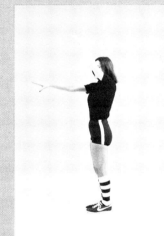

E Raise your left arm in an arc, up, over and behind. Straighten your knees as you raise your arm.

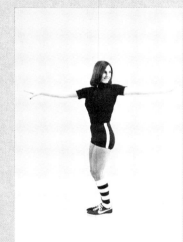

F Finish with your left palm up and your knees bent again.

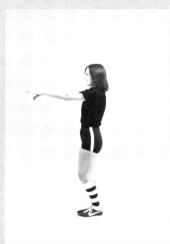

G Return to **A** by swinging your arm back the way it came, straightening and then bending your knees again.

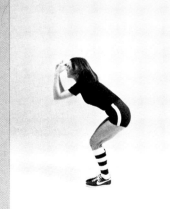

H Begin a downward swing by relaxing your neck, arms and upper body and bending your knees.

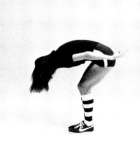

I Finish like this. Your head follows your arms down.

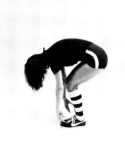

J Return to standing, uncurling smoothly.

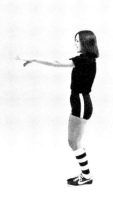

K Repeat, beginning with **B**.

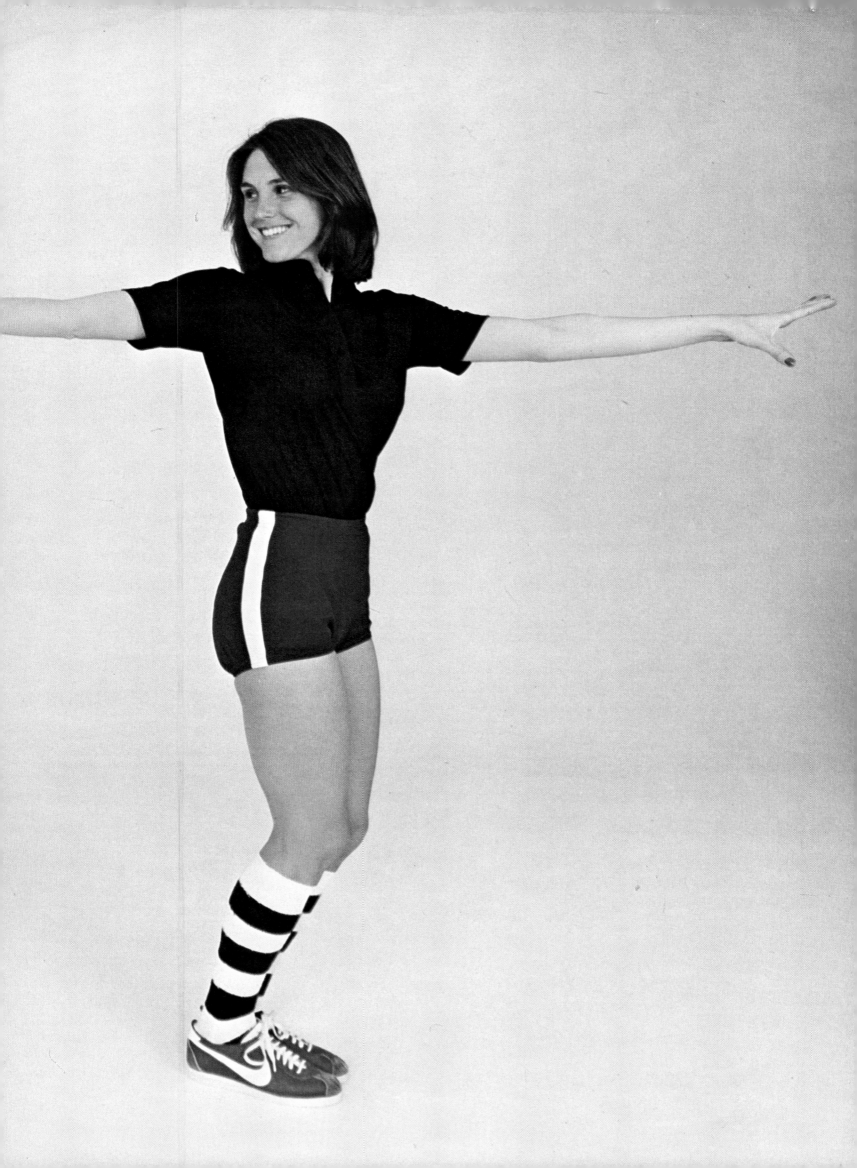

2 These shoulder twists strengthen the muscles in your shoulders and upper back. Hold your body upright by tightening your abdominal muscles as you perform the twists. Isolate your shoulders in your mind and twist them by rotating your whole arm and shoulder backward or forward. You begin with the palms of your hands facing the floor (A), but both palms should be facing upward at the end of each twist (B through E).

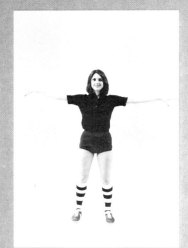

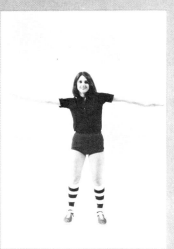

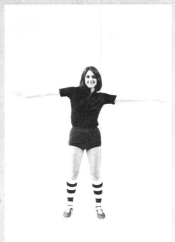

A Stand with your feet apart and your arms at shoulder height.

B Twist your right shoulder forward and your left backward.

C Twist your left shoulder forward and your right backward.

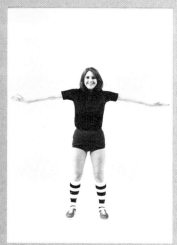

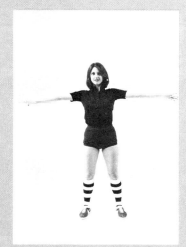

D Twist both shoulders forward together.

E Twist both shoulders backward together then repeat, beginning with **B.**

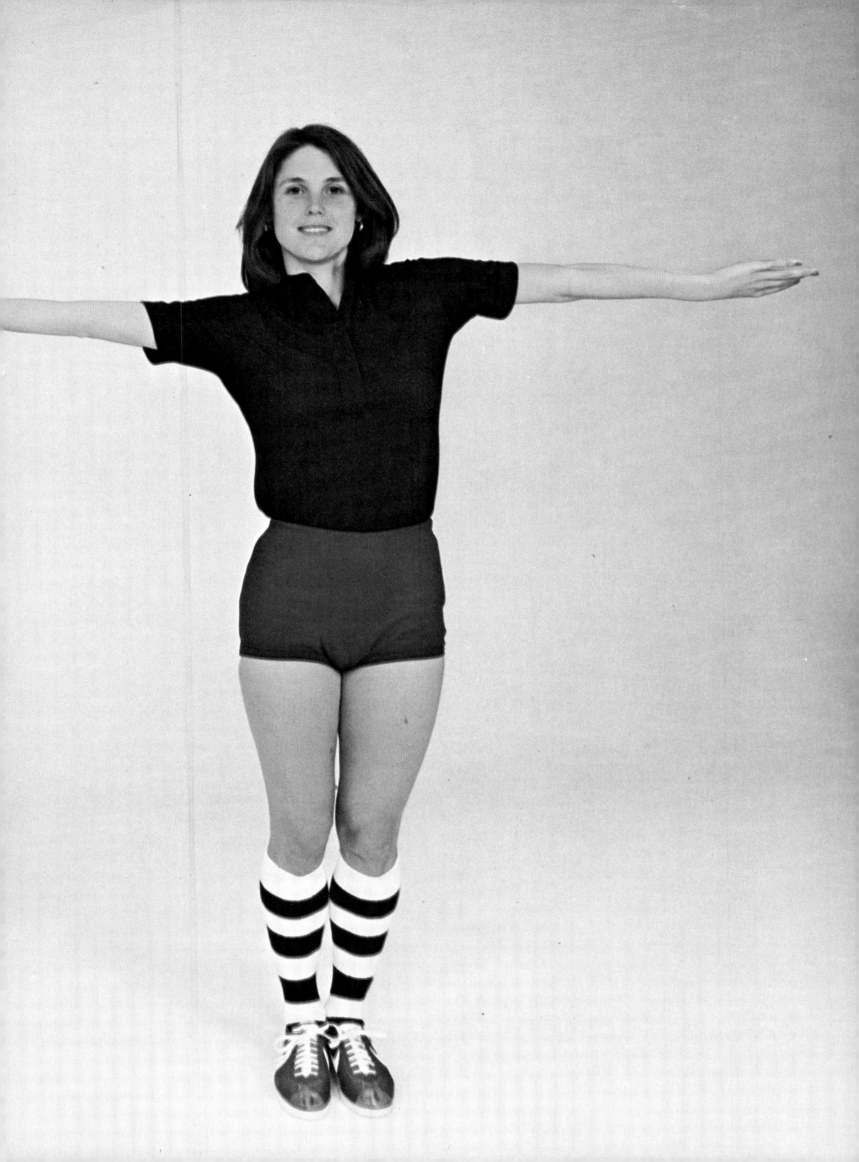

3 Frontal arm swings relax your arms following the last exercise as well as making your shoulders more flexible. Perform this sequence with a 'bouncing' motion (as in the first Movement Pattern) by bending your knees as your arms swing down and straightening them as your arms swing up. In the sequence shown you swing to the right, then left, then right again in a full circle. To repeat as mentioned in J, swing to the left, then right, then left again in a full circle.

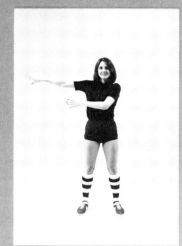

A Start with your arms left, like this, and your knees straight.

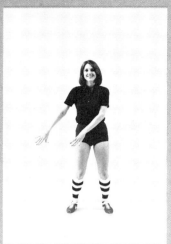

B Begin to swing right while bending your knees.

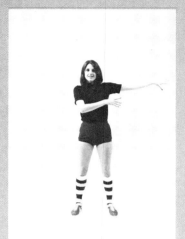

C Finish with your arms right and your knees straight.

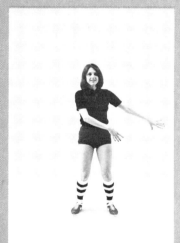

D Begin to swing left while bending your knees.

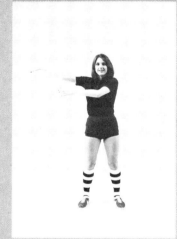

E Finish with your arms left and your knees straight.

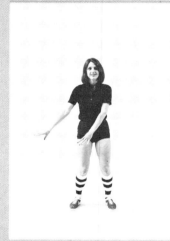

F Begin to swing right again while bending your knees.

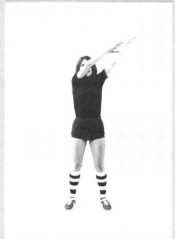

G Continue the swing to the right and up, in a circle over your head. Your knees are straight on the way up.

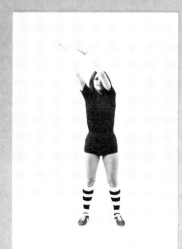

H Continue the swing in a circle over to the left and down, bending your knees as your arms come down.

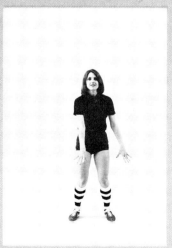

I Continue the swing down, with bent knees.

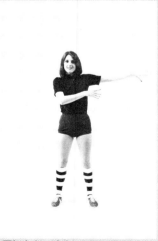

J Finish with your arms right and your knees straight. Repeat the entire sequence in the *opposite* direction.

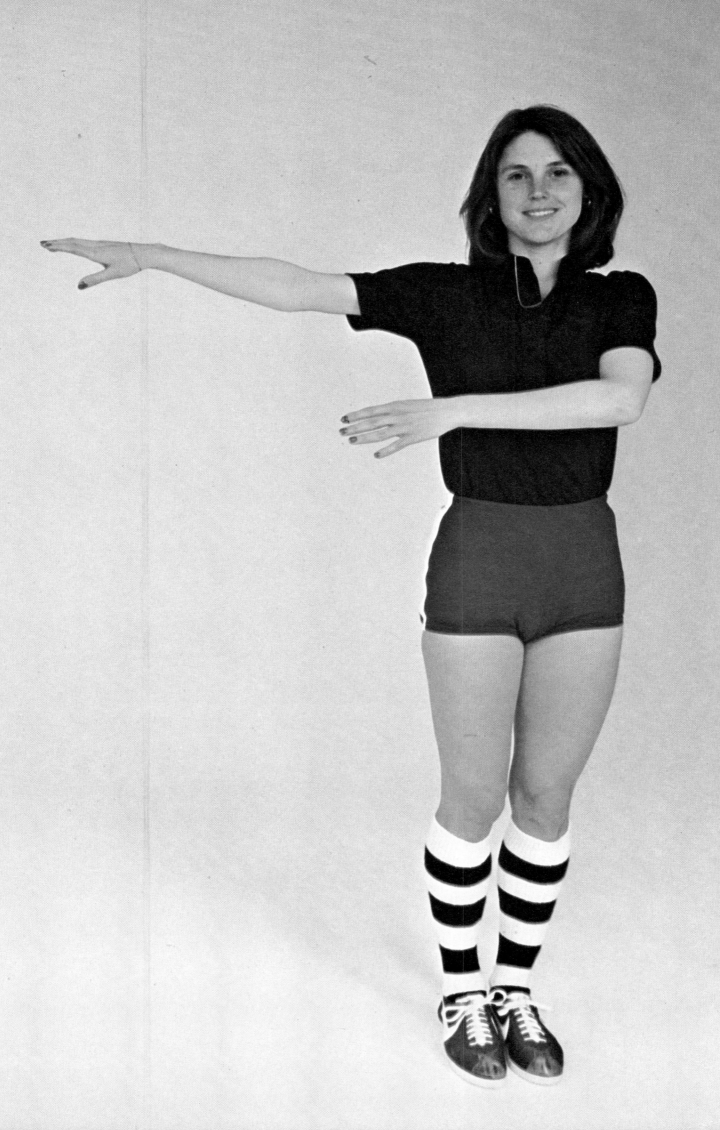

4 Pinching your shoulder blades together in this way stretches your upper chest and strengthens your shoulders and back. The positioning of your arms is important. Your forearms should be vertical, with your elbows in line with your hands. Make a smooth transition between each sequence. Be careful not to jerk your arms backward. Pull them gently.

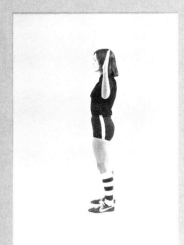 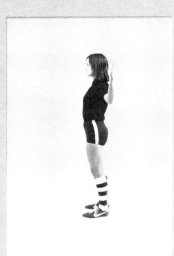 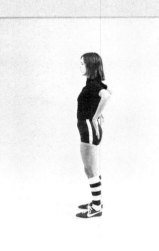

A Stand with your feet apart, both arms to the side at shoulder height with your elbows bent at 90°, and your hands up.

B Pull both arms and shoulders back to pinch your shoulder blades together twice.

C Lower your forearms with your hands pointing down. Pull your arms and shoulders back twice.

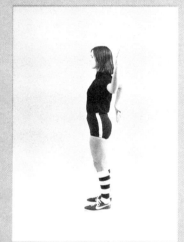 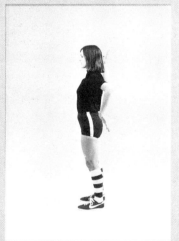

D Keeping your right arm in position **C**, move your left back to position **A**. Pull your arms and shoulders back twice.

E Reversing your arms, with the right up and the left down, pull back twice. Repeat, beginning with **B**.

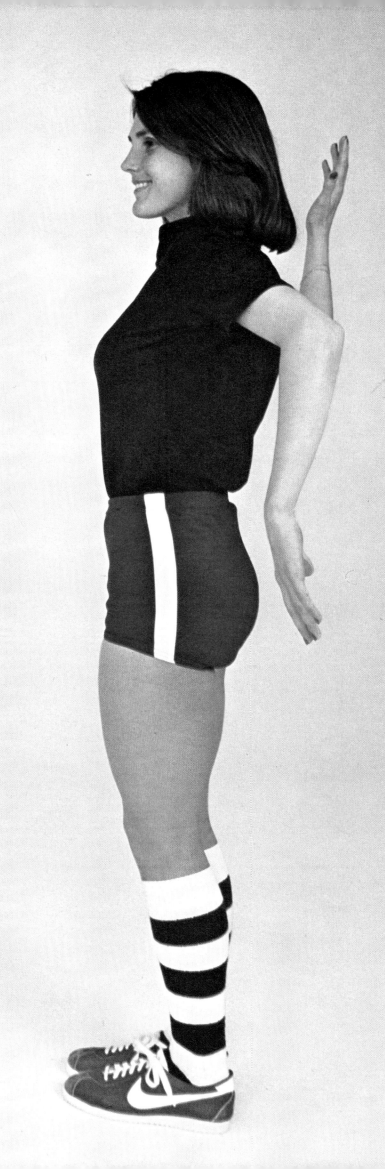

5 This simple Movement Pattern streamlines and strengthens your thighs and stretches your calves while improving your balance. It's also a good warm up for jogging. The secret of standing on one leg without falling over is to keep your eyes fixed on a spot on the wall or floor directly in front of you. In A and C you can feel the stretch in your thighs as you pull your heel in closer. In B and D you can feel the stretch in your calf and the force being exerted on the thigh of your bent leg.

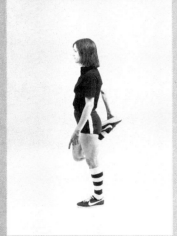 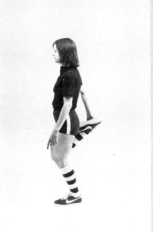 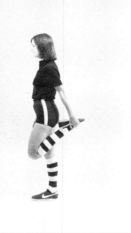 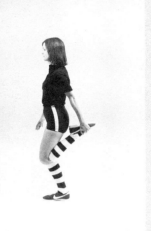

A Grasp your right foot in your right hand and pull it towards your buttocks.

B Bend and straighten your left knee slowly, at least five times.

C Grasp your left foot in your left hand and pull it towards your buttocks.

D Bend and straighten your right knee slowly, at least five times. Change legs as in **A** and repeat, beginning with **B.**

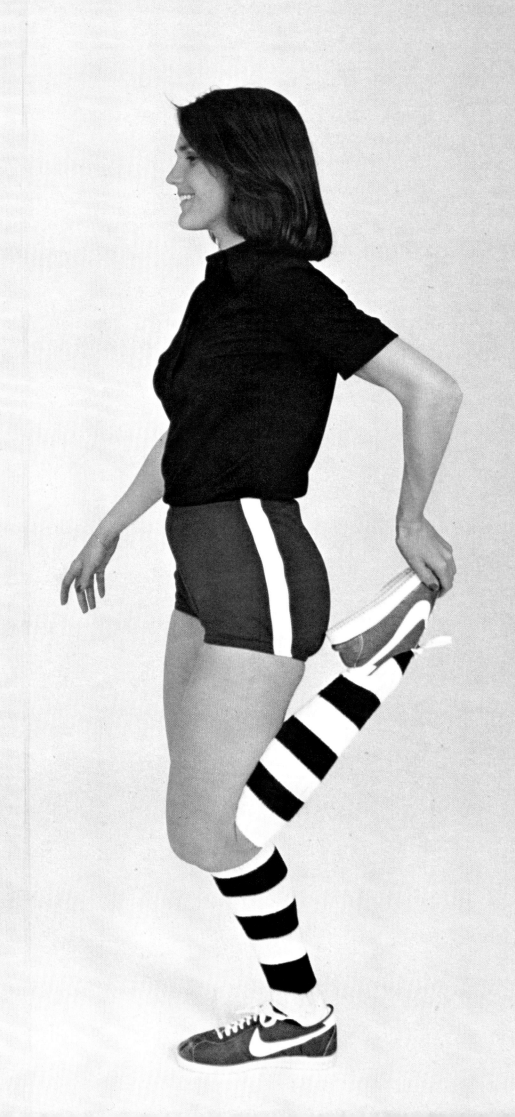

6 This Movement Pattern tests your balance and coordination. It consists of knee lifts with waist twists which improve your hip flexibility and thigh strength while firming and slimming your waist. As with all the Movement Patterns, try to give your facial muscles a workout with a smile. In B and D your raised leg should be at your side, not to the front. Do this by turning your hip out as you raise your leg.

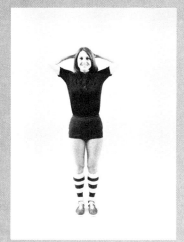

A Stand with your feet slightly apart and your hands clasped behind your head.

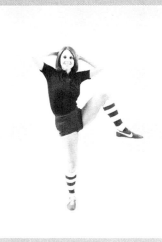

B Lift your right knee toward your right elbow.

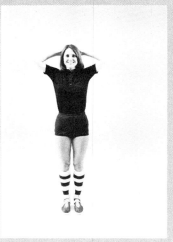

C Return to the floor as in **A**.

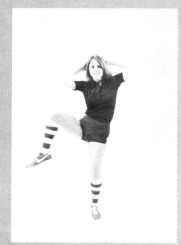

D Lift your left knee toward your left elbow.

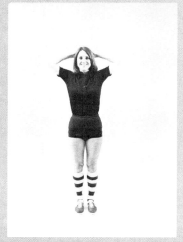

E Return to the floor.

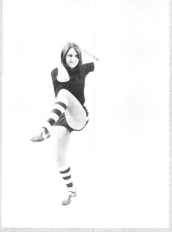

F Twist your right knee up toward your left elbow.

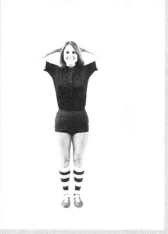

G Return to the floor.

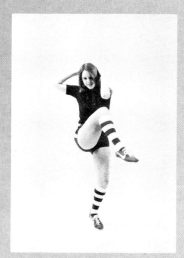

H Twist your left knee up toward your right elbow.

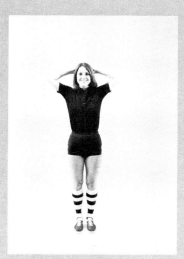

I Return to the floor and repeat, beginning with **B**.

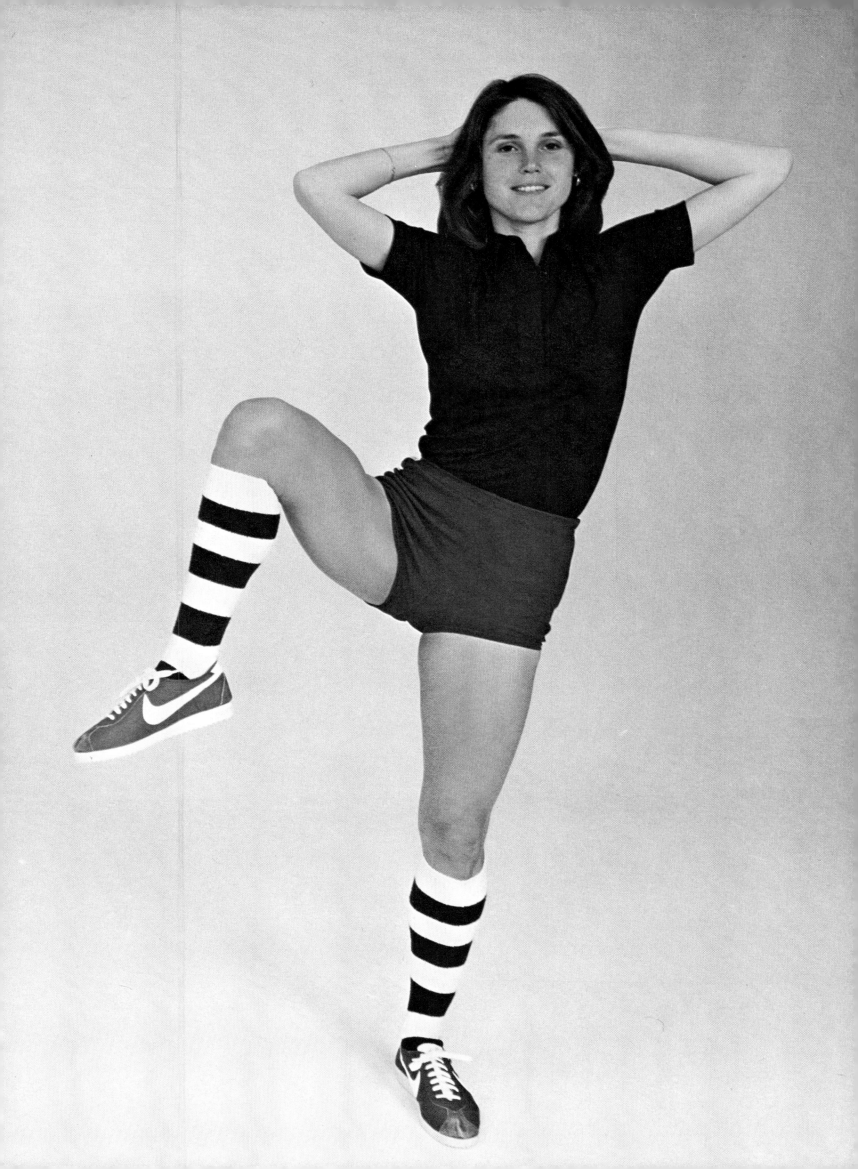

7 This Movement Pattern stretches your hamstrings (the muscles in the back of your thigh) as you slowly straighten each leg. It also firms your buttocks and is a good stretching exercise to use before and after running or jogging. Straighten your legs only as far as comfortable and concentrate on keeping your weight on your *straight* leg, keeping the other one bent. Your hands may lift slightly off the floor in B and D as you straighten your leg.

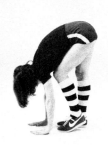

A Crouch with your hands on the floor.

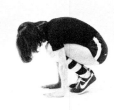

B Place your weight over your right leg and slowly straighten up, keeping your left knee bent.

C Relax as in **A**.

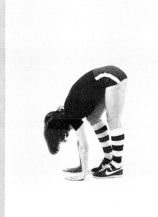

D Place your weight over your left leg and slowly straighten up, keeping your right knee bent.

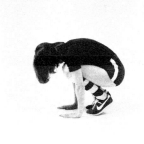

E Relax as in **A** and then repeat, beginning with **B**.

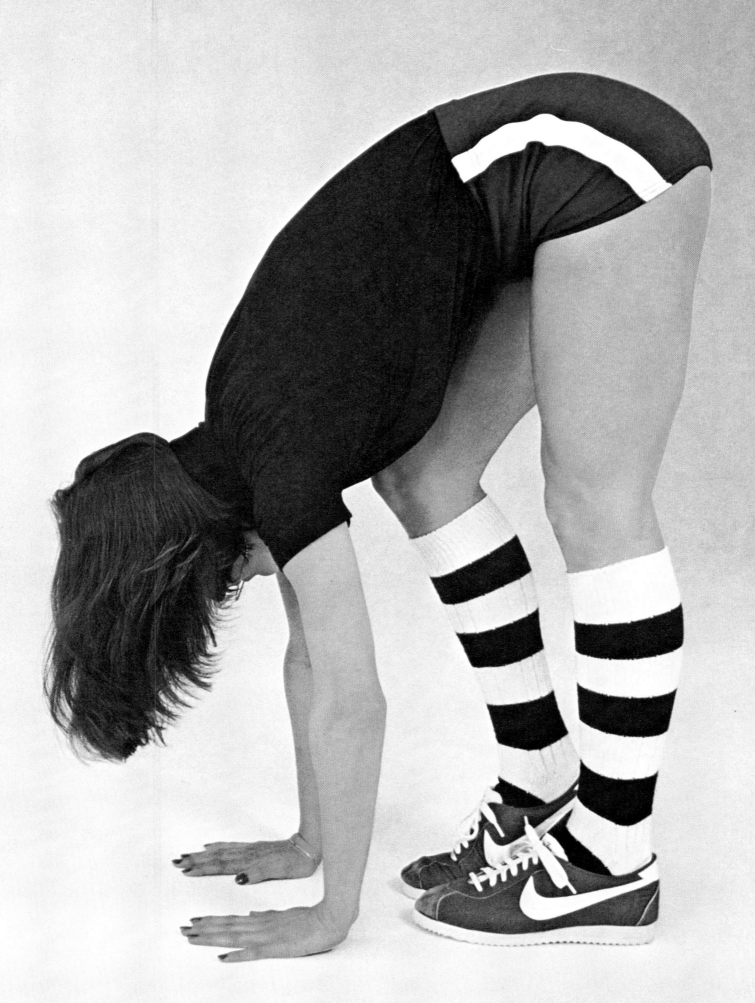

8 As well as stretching your hamstrings, this Movement Pattern strengthens your shoulders and upper back muscles. Try to keep your back flat in C as you raise your arms. Uncurl smoothly from D to E, bringing your head up last.

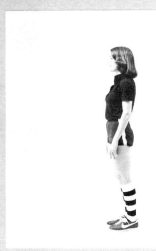

A Stand with your feet together.

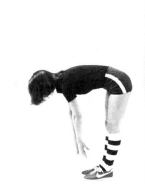

B Bend forward from the waist, with your back horizontal and your arms hanging loosely.

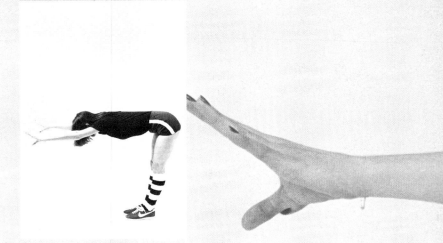

C Slowly raise your arms and reach forward.

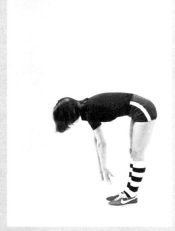

D Lower your arms as in **B**.

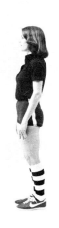

E Slowly uncurl upward to **A** and repeat, beginning with **B**.

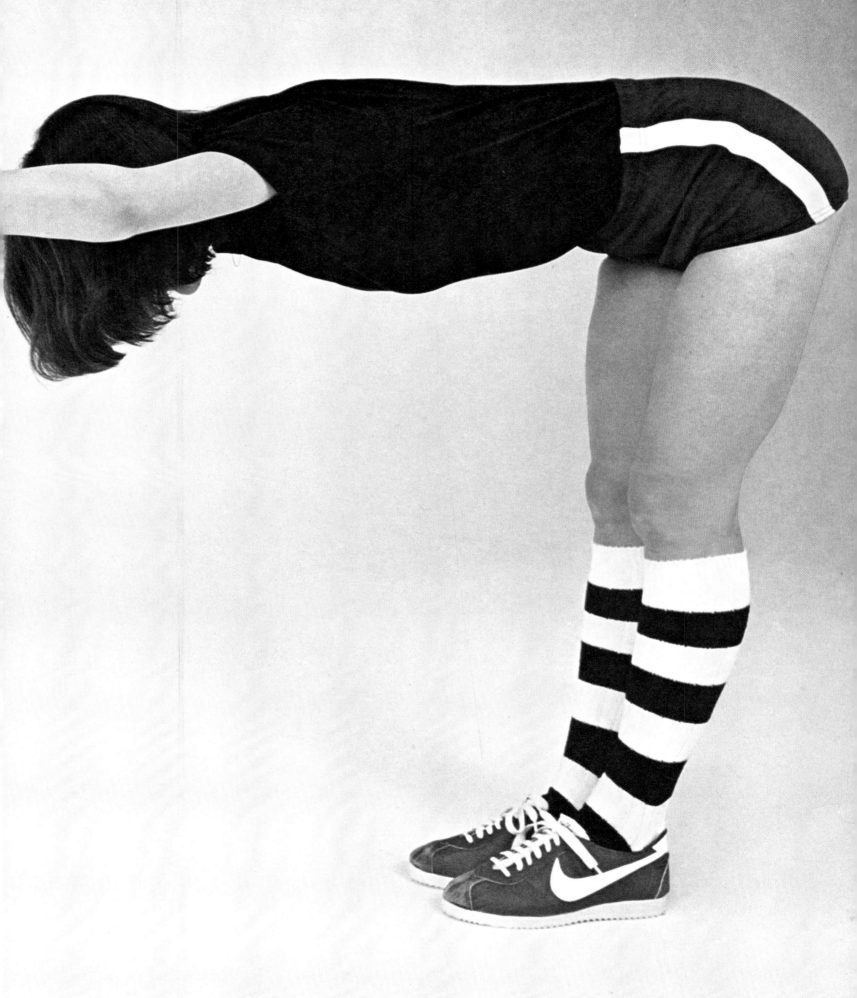

9 This Movement Pattern has several benefits. It strengthens your thighs, firms your buttocks and improves your hip flexibility. The body swings are relaxing and involve the coordination of your arms and legs. From D to L your arms move with your legs—circle them down as you lower your hips and circle them up as you push off to stand. Turn your toes out slightly in E and J to help in lowering your hips.

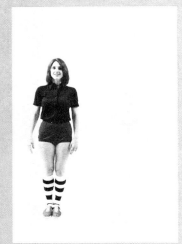

A Stand with your feet together.

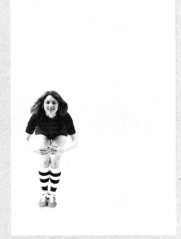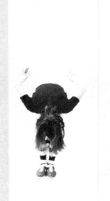

B Bend your knees and swing down with your head following your arms.

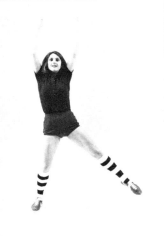

C Finish like this, with your neck relaxed.

D Straighten up with your head following your arms and move your right leg to the right.

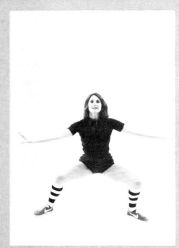

E Bend your knees, lower your hips and circle your arms down and to the sides.

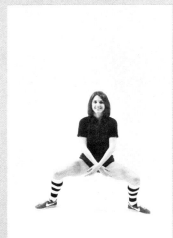

F Finish like this with your arms crossed and your weight distributed evenly on both feet.

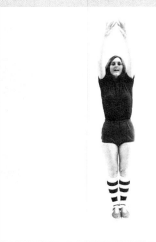

G Push off from your right leg and straighten up by bringing your legs together and circling your arms to the sides and up.

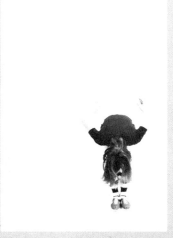

H Swing down as in **B** and **C**.

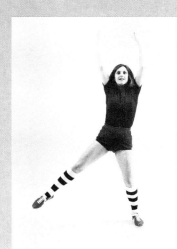

I Straighten up with your head following your arms and move your left leg to the left.

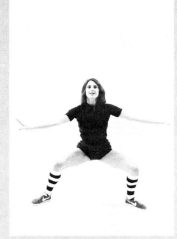

J Bend your knees, lower your hips and swing your arms down and to the sides.

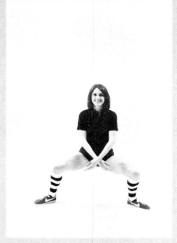

K Finish as in **F**.

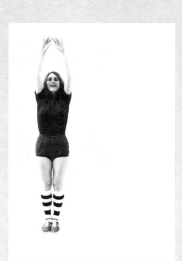

L Push off from your left leg and straighten up as in **G**. Repeat the sequence, beginning with **B**.

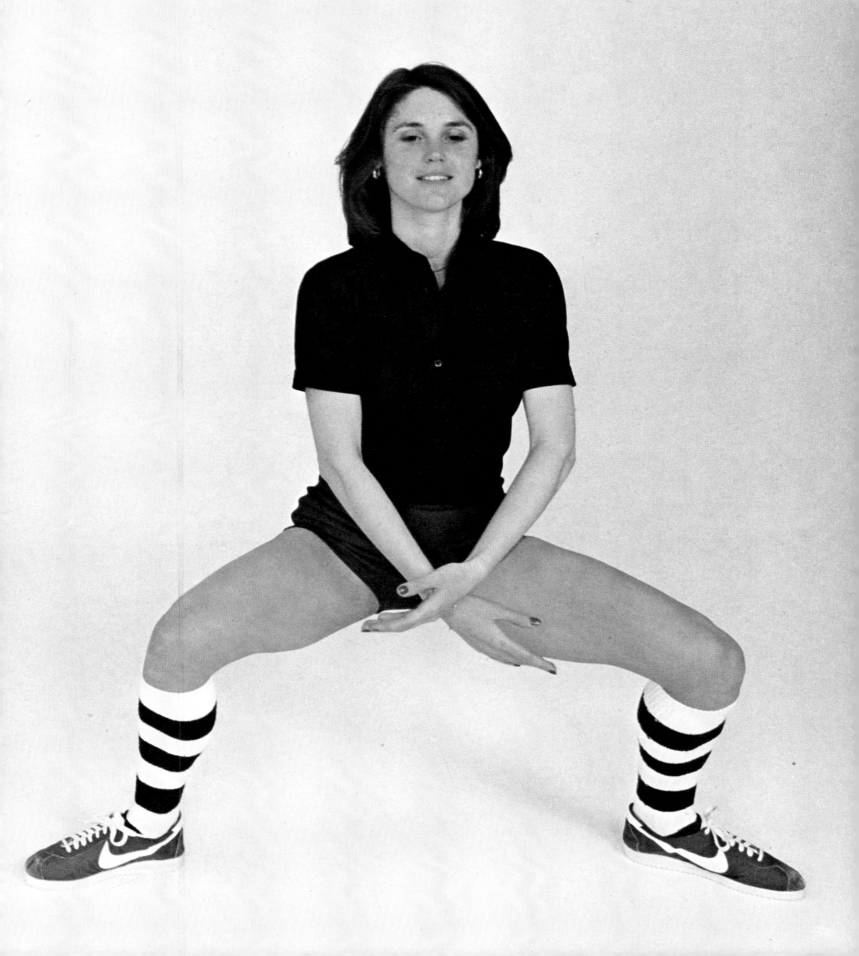

10 Alternate toe touching stretches and strengthens your thighs and rotates your shoulders for improved flexibility. To master the side to side movement, bend one knee and shift your weight over it, then bend the other knee and shift your weight over it, shifting continuously from side to side. Accompany this with your opposite arm reaching across your bent knee to touch the floor beyond your toe, and your other arm stretching overhead.

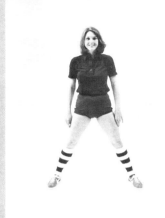

A Stand with your feet wide apart.

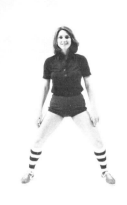

B Bend your knees slightly.

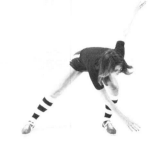

C Bend your right knee, then shift your weight over it and reach your left arm across your right leg.

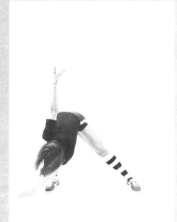

D Bend your left knee, then shift your weight over it and reach your right arm across your left leg.

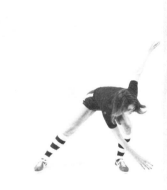

E Repeat, beginning with **C**. Continue back and forth between **C** and **D**.

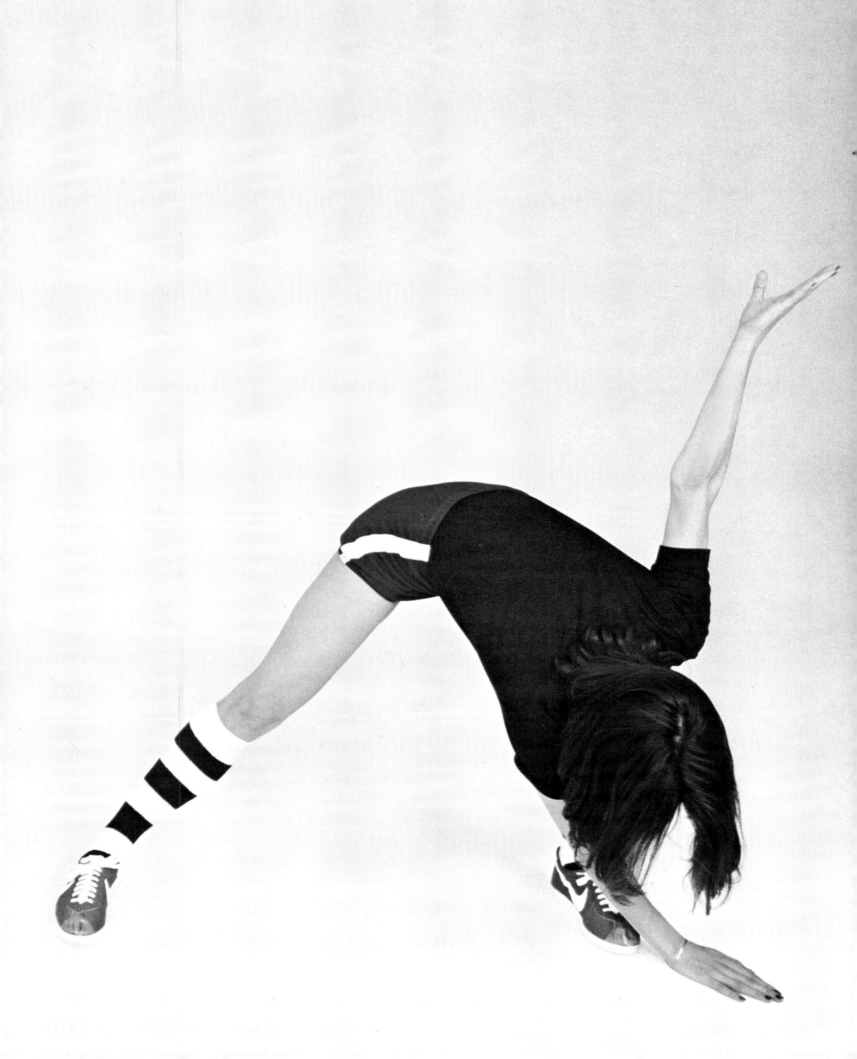

11 This Movement Pattern is very much like 10 and provides similar benefits. The same procedure is followed, shifting your weight from side to side over your bent knee. The important difference is that your opposite arm reaches across to your *straight* leg as opposed to your bent leg in 10. This stretches the muscles in the back of your thigh. Touch the toe of your straight leg with the hand of your opposite arm. Swing back and forth between C and D from four to twelve times.

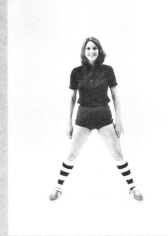

A Stand with your feet wide apart.

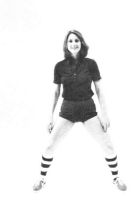

B Bend your knees slightly.

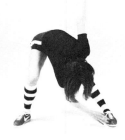

C Bend your left knee, then shift your weight over it, and reach your left arm across to touch your right toe.

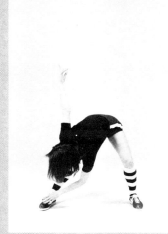

D Bend your right knee, then shift your weight over it, and reach your right arm across to touch your left toe.

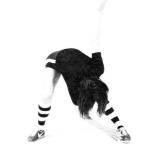

E Repeat, beginning with **C**. Continue back and forth between **C** and **D**.

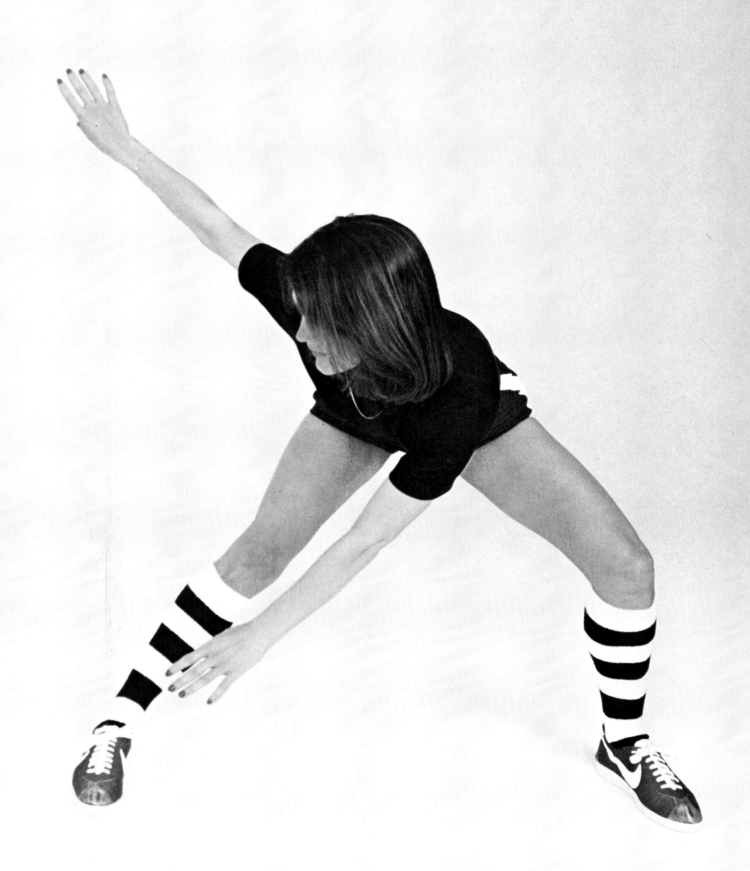

Relax

After the efforts of the previous Movement Patterns, this deep breathing and body swing exercise relaxes your muscles and gives you renewed energy. In B and E you should keep your back flat and your head up. In C and D close your eyes and concentrate on relaxing all your muscles. Exhale deeply as you 'collapse' in C and D and inhale as you uncurl up to E. Repeat this sequence until you feel rested and ready to continue.

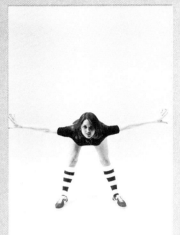

A Bend forward with your arms wide and upper body parallel to the floor.

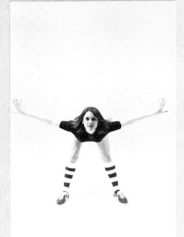

B Maintain position **A** and press your chest toward the floor.

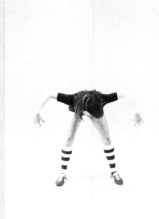

C Relax the pressure, bend your knees and begin to 'collapse' your upper body to the floor.

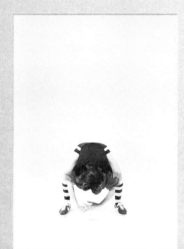

D Finish in a slump like this. Hold for a few seconds.

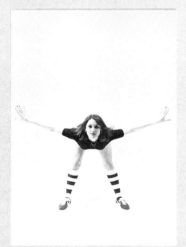

E Uncurl to **A** and repeat, beginning with **B**.

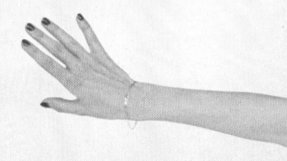

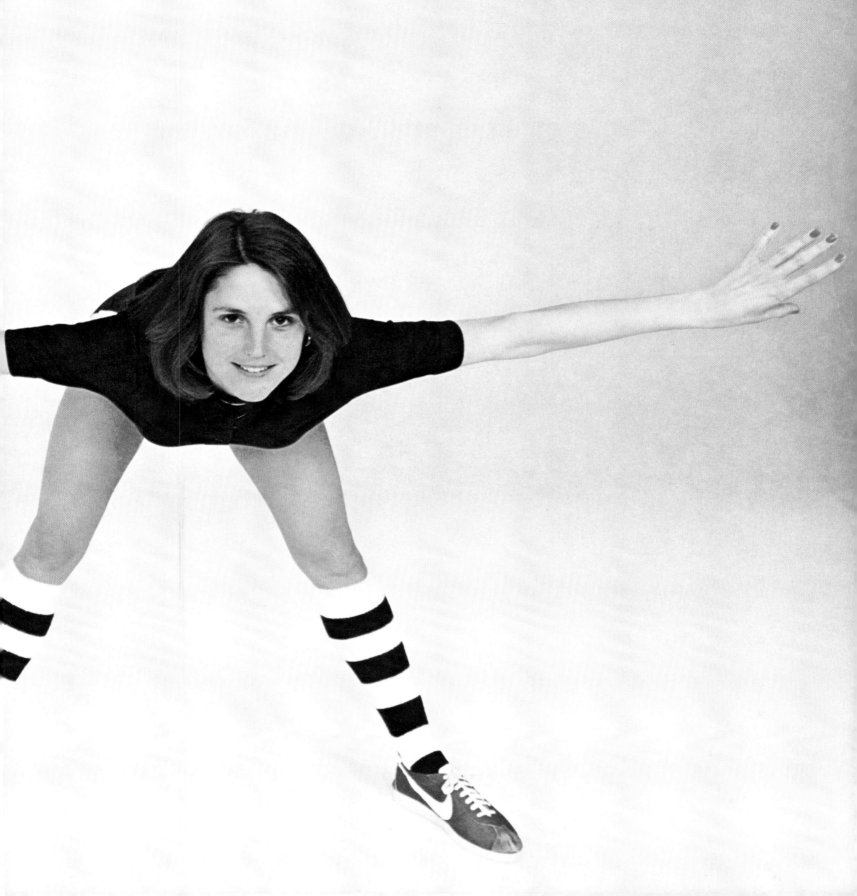

12 The next series of Movement Patterns is performed from a kneeling position. This one strengthens your thigh and abdominal muscles. In C you can feel your thighs doing the work as they hold your weight, while your abdominal muscles hold the angle of your body.

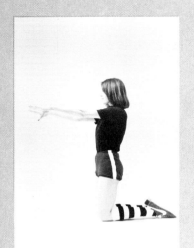

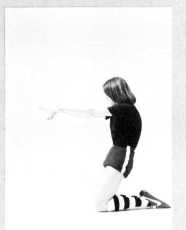

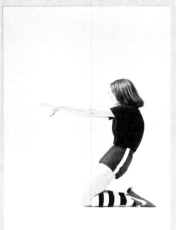

A Kneel with your back straight and your arms at shoulder height.

B Tuck your chin to your chest, round your shoulders slightly forward and pull your stomach in.

C Slowly lean back and hold for a few seconds.

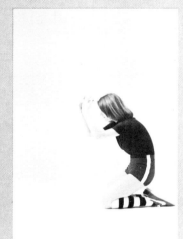

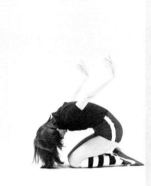

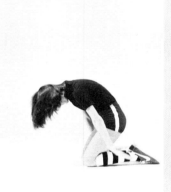

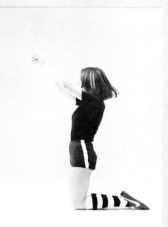

D Relax your neck, arms and upper body and begin to swing down.

E Finish the swing like this. Your head goes down last.

F Dropping your arms, slowly uncurl. Bring your head up last.

G Straighten your arms and upper body to this position then repeat, beginning with **B**.

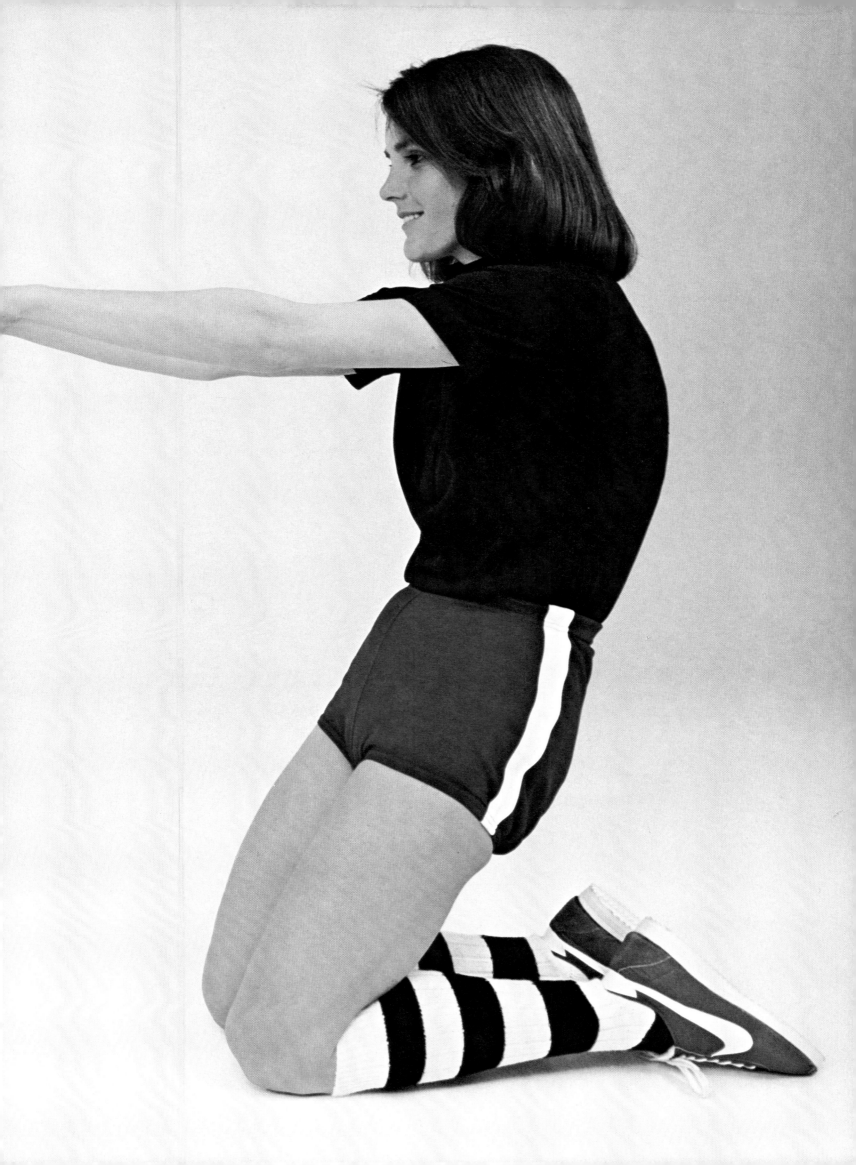

13 The twisting action of your waist, while kneeling, helps to slim your waistline while strengthening your thighs. Your back is stretched when you bend forward and strengthened when you lift up. These manoeuvres also help to improve your balance. In C and G let your elbow guide your head and neck downward only as far as comfortable. Keep your upper body vertical when you straighten up in E and I — don't let it arch backward. Perform the sequence smoothly and rhythmically.

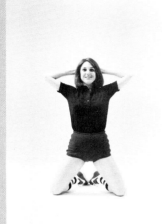

A Kneel with your legs shoulder width apart and your hands behind your head.

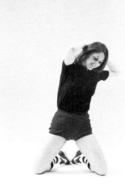

B Bend forward and down, twisting your left elbow toward your right knee.

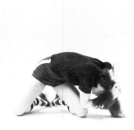

C Finish with your left elbow touching your right knee.

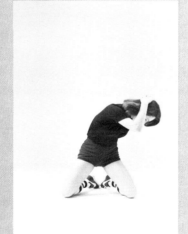

D Slowly straighten up the way you came down.

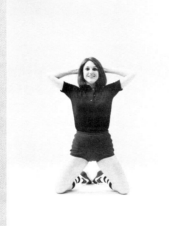

E Finish like this.

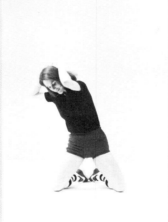

F Bend forward and down, twisting your right elbow toward your left knee.

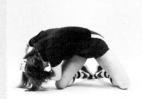

G Finish with your right elbow touching your left knee.

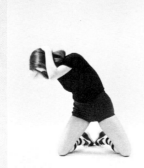

H Slowly straighten up the way you came down.

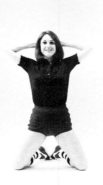

I Finish in this position. Then repeat, beginning with **B.**

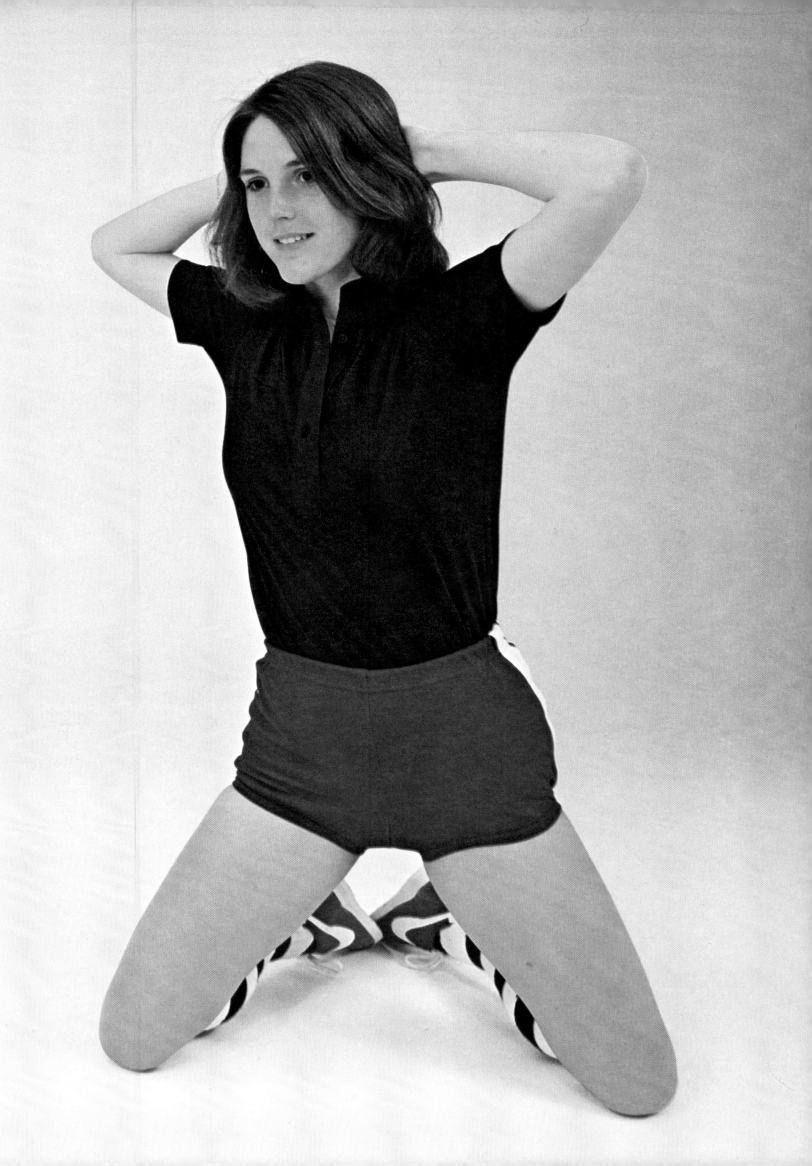

14 Side stretches help to slim your waist, and these stretch the inner thigh of your straight leg as well. You should feel the stretches if you are doing them properly. When stretching to the sides keep your back straight and your shoulders over your hips to avoid twisting forward or backward. Stretch to the side only as far as comfortable in B and G and press gently. Keep up your momentum between the side stretches and the down swing.

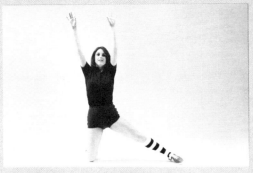

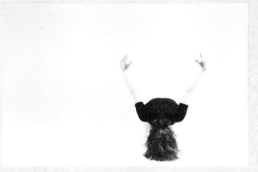

A Kneel on your left knee with your right leg extended to the right and your arms overhead.

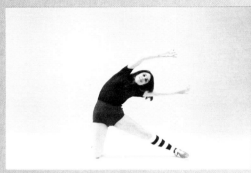

B Stretch to the right over your right leg, then gently press twice with your upper body.

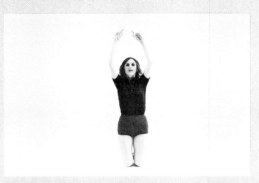

C Straighten up, bringing in your right knee to join your left, and begin to swing down.

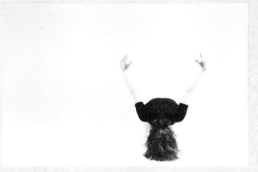

D Finish the swing like this. Your head comes down last.

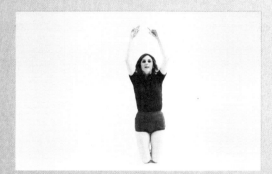

E Slowly uncurl, bringing your head up last. Finish with your arms overhead.

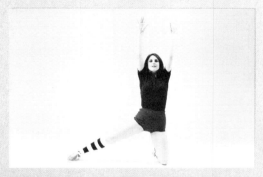

F Extend your left leg to the left.

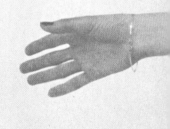

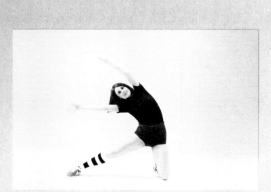

G Stretch over your left leg and gently press twice with your upper body.

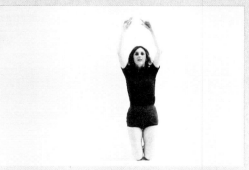

H Straighten up, bringing in your left knee to join your right. To continue, swing down then up as in **D** and **E**. Repeat beginning with **A**.

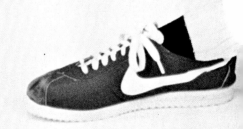

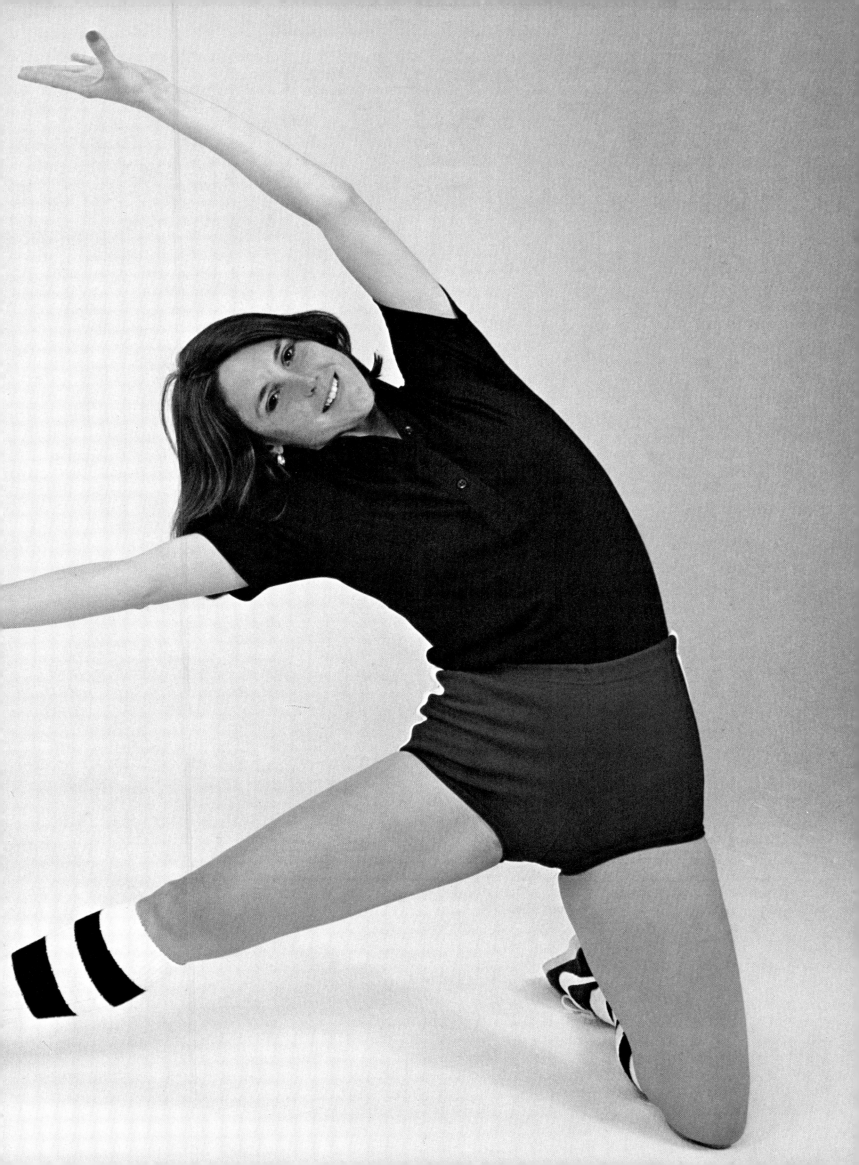

15 The symmetry of this sequence makes it very satisfying to perform. It stretches your hamstring muscles and improves the flexibility of your hips. Make sure your legs are a comfortable distance apart. When assuming positions A and F extend your leg to the side of your body, not to the front or back. Your hips should face the direction of the movement.

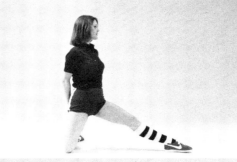

A Kneel on your left knee and face your extended right leg. Clasp your hands behind your back.

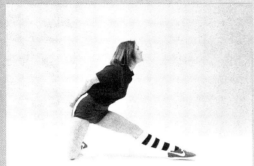

B Slowly lower your upper body down over your right leg.

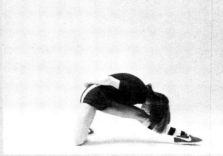

C Finish like this, with your head coming down last.

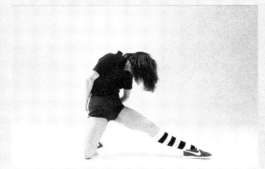

D Slowly uncurl.

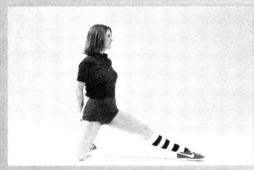

E Finish as in **A**, and repeat from four to twelve times, beginning with **B**.

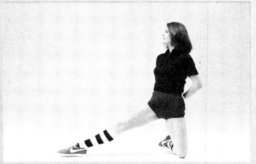

F Kneel on your right knee and face your extended left leg. Clasp your hands behind your back.

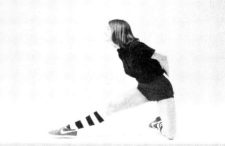

G Slowly lower your upper body down over your left leg.

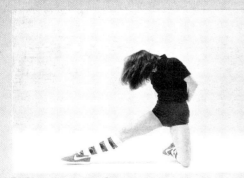

I Slowly uncurl.

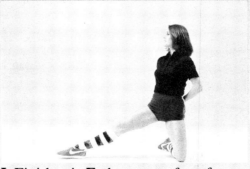

J Finish as in **F**, then repeat from four to twelve times, beginning with **G**.

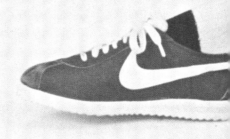

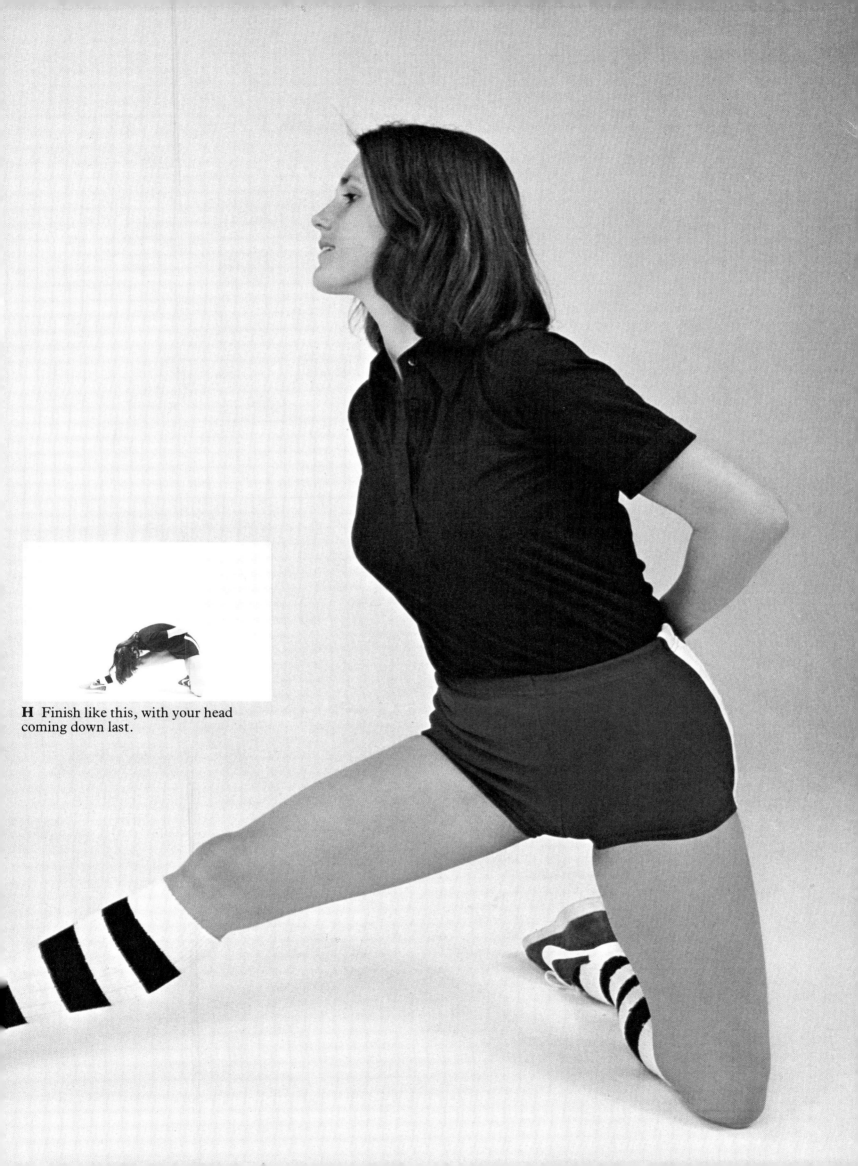

H Finish like this, with your head coming down last.

16 In the beginning it will be tiring to hold your leg aloft in this way, but your thighs, hips and buttocks are all strengthened by it. Rest if you feel too much strain. To help keep your back straight and to maintain your balance, fix your eyes on a spot in front of you or on the floor between your hands.

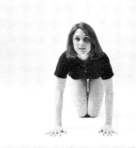

A Rest on your hands and knees.

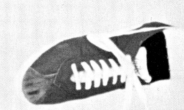

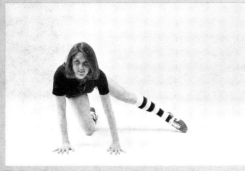

E Lower and raise your leg twice.

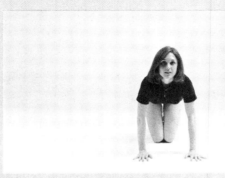

F Rest on your hands and knees.

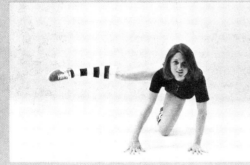

G Extend your left leg horizontally to the left.

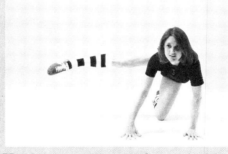

H Make a small circle forward with your leg twice.

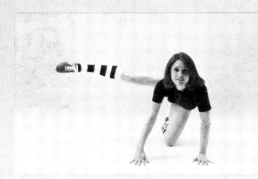

I Make a small circle backward twice.

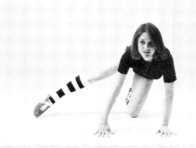

J Lower and raise your leg twice.

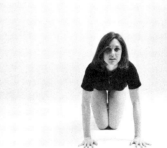

K Resume position **A** and repeat, beginning with **B**.

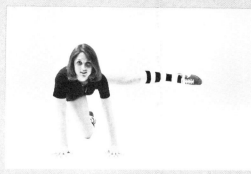

B Extend your right leg horizontally to the right.

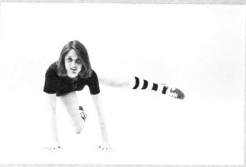

C Make a small circle forward with your leg twice.

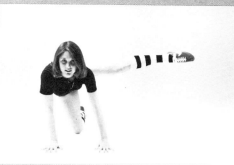

D Make a small circle backward twice.

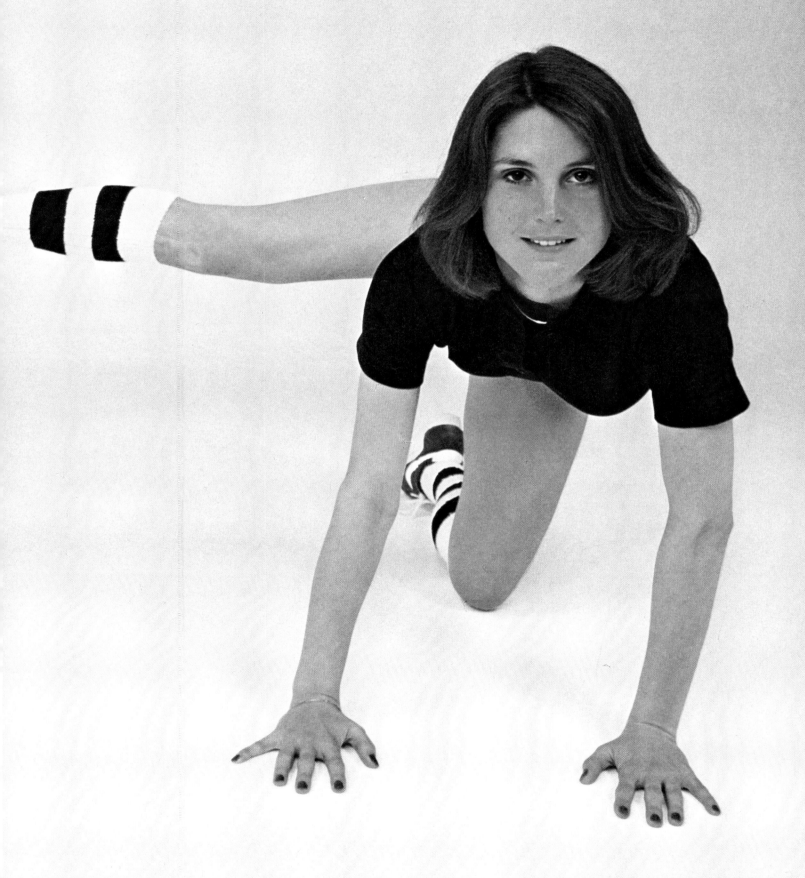

17 The next three Movement Patterns begin from a prone position. This one strengthens the hamstring muscles in the back of your thighs and firms your buttocks. To avoid straining your lower back make sure your hips don't come off the floor and don't raise your leg too high. You should repeat each leg raise from four to twelve times before repeating with the other leg.

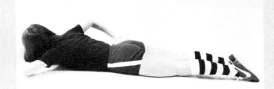

A Put your left hand under your chin and your right hand under your right hip.

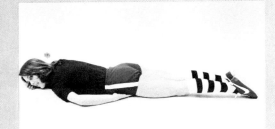

D Put your right hand under your chin and your left hand under your left hip.

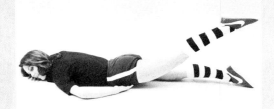

E Lock your left knee, press your hip into your hand and raise your left leg slowly.

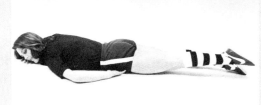

F Lower your leg slowly. Continue to raise and lower it to complete your sequence.

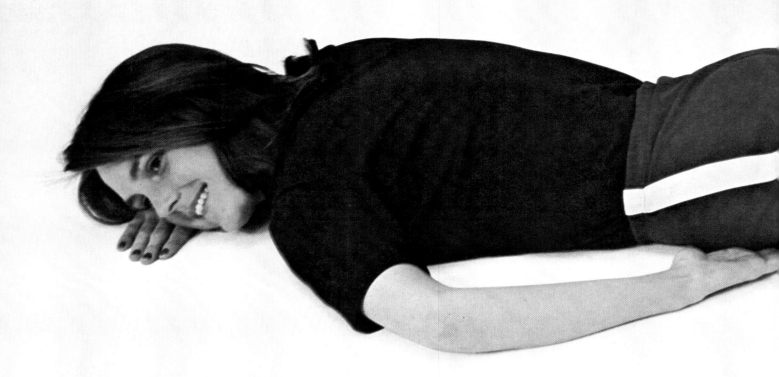

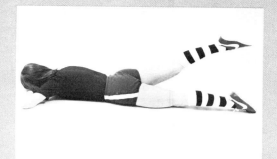 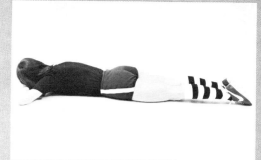

B Lock your right knee, press your hip into your hand and raise your right leg slowly.

C Lower your leg slowly. Continue to raise and lower it to complete your sequence.

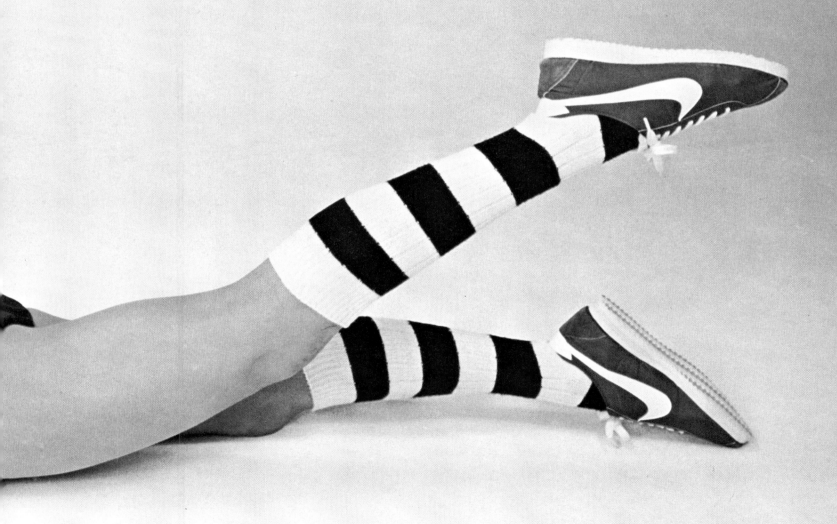

18 This Movement Pattern strengthens your neck, arms, and upper back, as well as your legs and buttocks. When raising your head and shoulders in B and F push up with your arms — don't lift with your back — and keep your elbows on the floor. Your hips should remain on the floor when raising your legs in D and H. Try to achieve a rhythmical rocking motion (without involving your back) throughout the sequence.

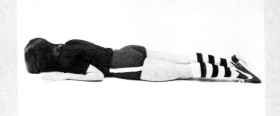

A Lie with your hands under your shoulders and your elbows on the floor.

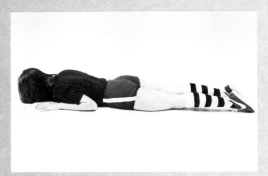

E Slowly lower your leg to the floor.

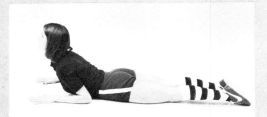

F Slowly push your head and shoulders up from the floor as in **B**.

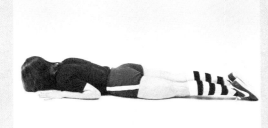

G Slowly lower to the floor.

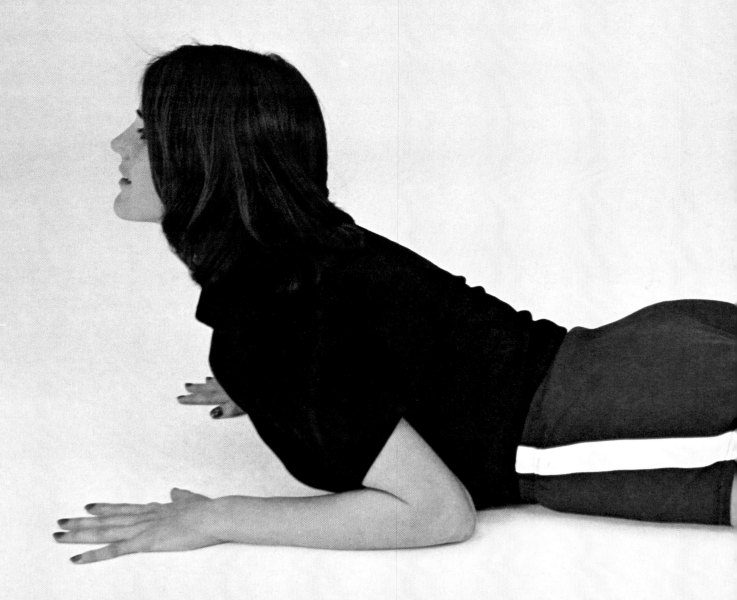

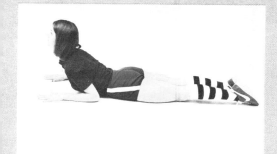

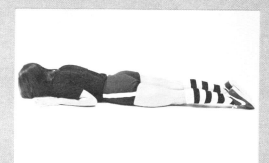

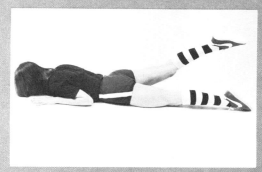

B Slowly push your head and shoulders up from the floor.

C Slowly lower to the floor.

D Lock your knee and slowly raise your right leg, keeping your hip on the floor.

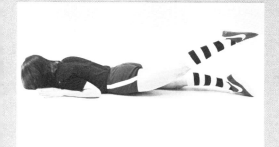

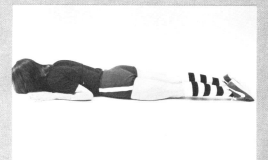

H Lock your knee and slowly raise your left leg, keeping your hip on the floor.

I Slowly lower to the floor and repeat, beginning with **B.**

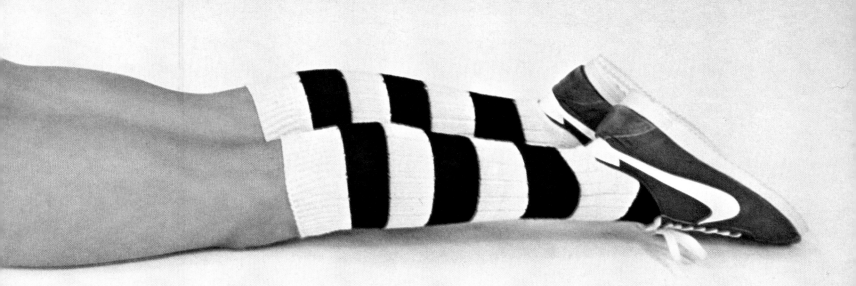

19 Push ups with accompanying leg lifts strengthen your upper arms, shoulders and abdominal muscles. Concentrate on keeping your back straight—don't arch it—and try to keep your leg parallel to the floor when raising and lowering it. Perform this sequence at a fairly brisk pace.

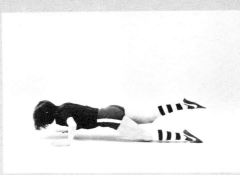

A Lie with your hands under your shoulders and elbows up.

B Push up and back with your arms while raising your right leg.

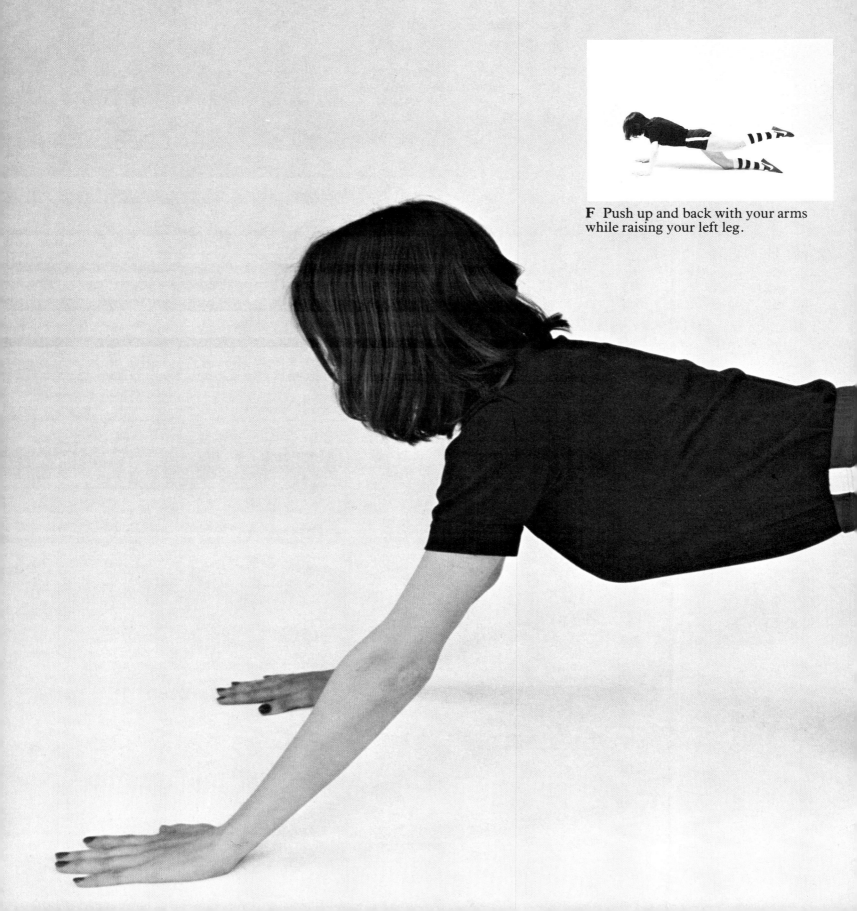

F Push up and back with your arms while raising your left leg.

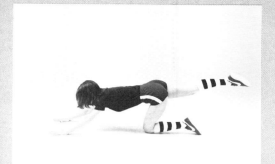

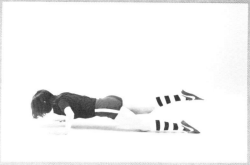

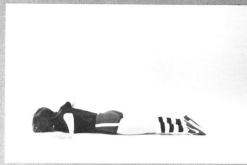

C Finish with your arms extended and your right leg parallel to the floor.

D Lower back to the floor the way you came up.

E Resume position **A**.

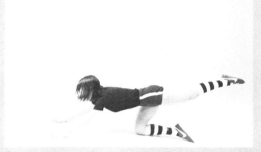

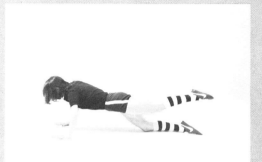

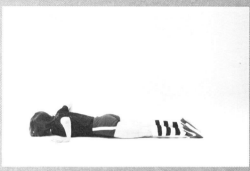

G Finish with your arms extended and your left leg parallel to the floor.

H Lower back to the floor the way you came up.

I Resume position **A** then repeat, beginning with **B**.

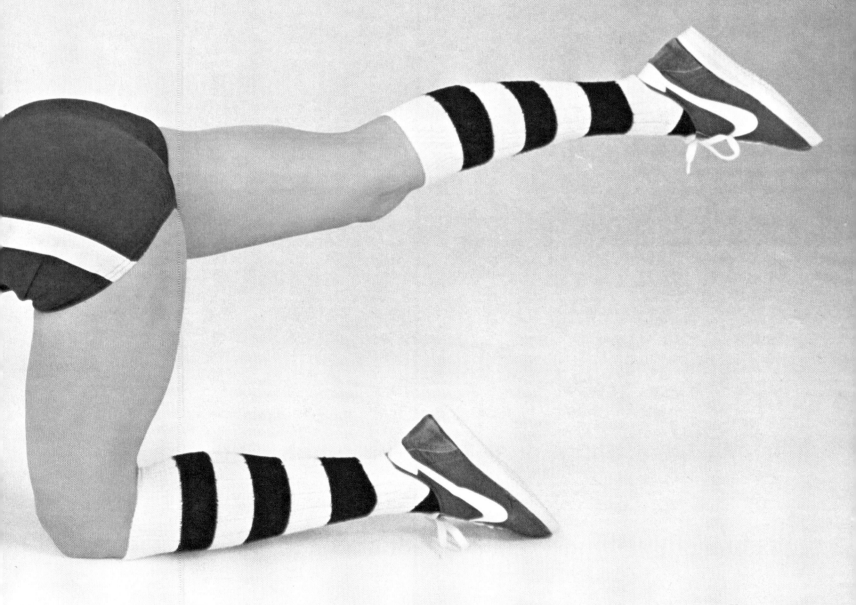

20 This special aerobic sequence is designed to accelerate your heart rate to improve your cardiovascular fitness and stamina. You should spend at least three minutes on this Movement Pattern, about 30 seconds on each different position. Begin slowly in A and B, then accelerate your pace for the other sequences. Slow down again in K. In I and J your head and shoulders face forward.

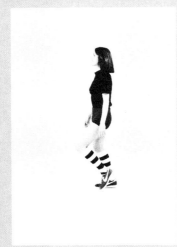

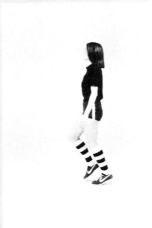

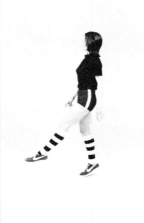

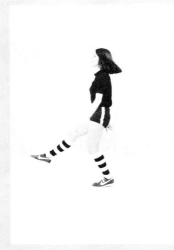

A Run lightly on the spot with your arms and upper body relaxed.

B Continue running for 30 seconds.

C Kick forward with straight legs.

D Continue kicking for 30 seconds.

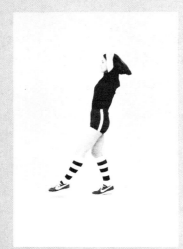

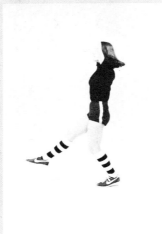

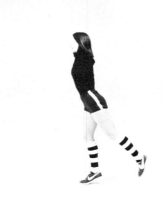

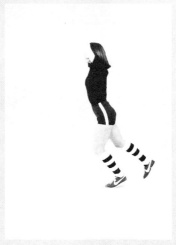

E Continue kicking and raise your hands above your head.

F Continue this way for 30 seconds.

G Kick backward with straight legs with your arms overhead.

H Continue this way for 30 seconds.

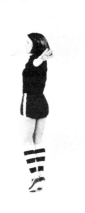

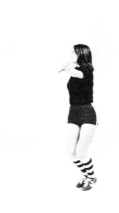

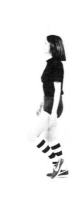

I Lower your arms to shoulder height. Twist at the waist and hop right and left, with your feet together.

J Continue twisting and hopping for 30 seconds.

K Relax your upper body and run lightly on the spot as in **A** and **B** for 30 seconds.

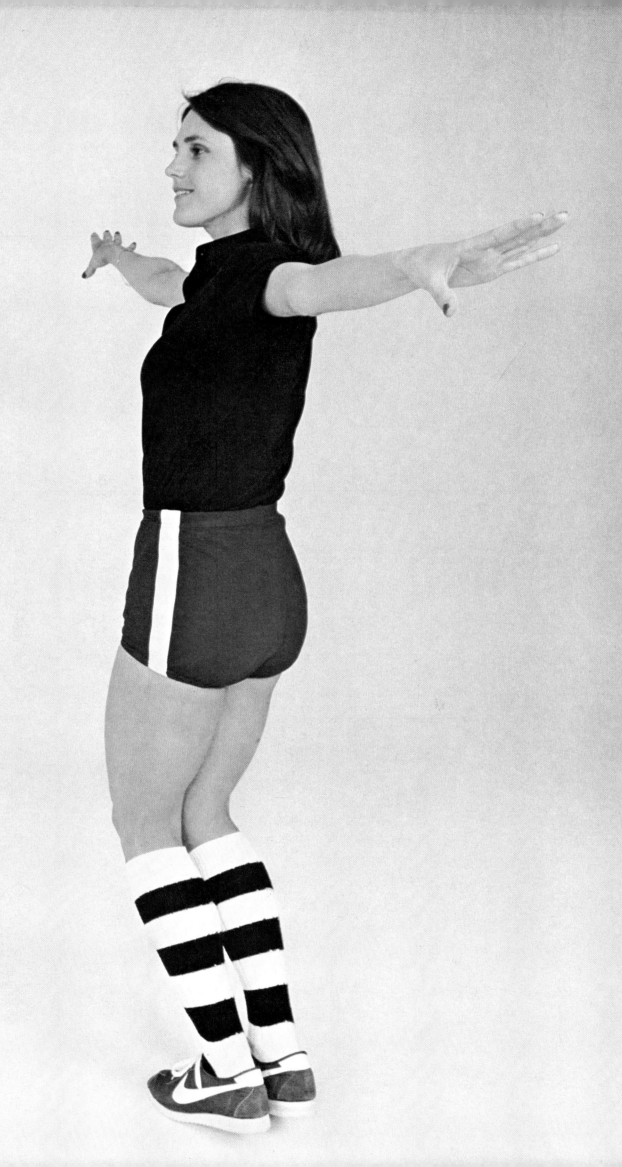

Relax

These deep breathing movements help you to recover your energy by supplying more oxygen to your body while you are in a relaxed state. Concentrate on breathing deeply—always inhale as you lift your arms and shoulders and exhale as you lower them. Perform this sequence in a continuous movement until you feel rested.

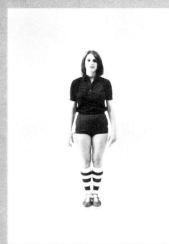

A Relax completely, standing with your feet together and your arms loosely at your sides.

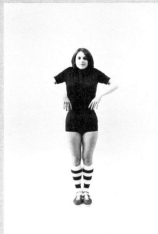

B Rotate your shoulders forward, up, back and down in an imaginary circle around your neck.

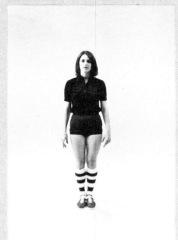

C Return to **A.**

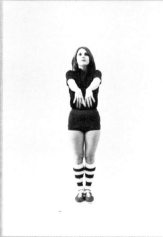

D Begin to raise your arms upward in an arc. Inhale deeply.

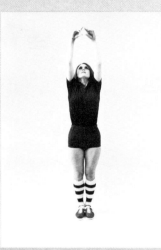

E Finish the arc with your arms overhead. Continue to inhale.

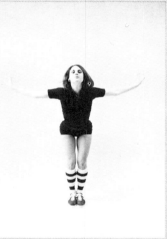

F Bending your knees slightly, let your arms fall as you relax your upper body in a downward swing. Exhale deeply.

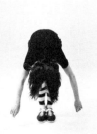

G Finish the swing with your knees bent, your body limp, your eyes closed and all the air expelled from your lungs.

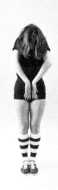

H Breathing in, uncurl smoothly to a vertical position, bringing your head and shoulders up last.

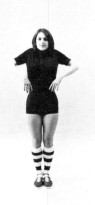

I Repeat, beginning with **B.**

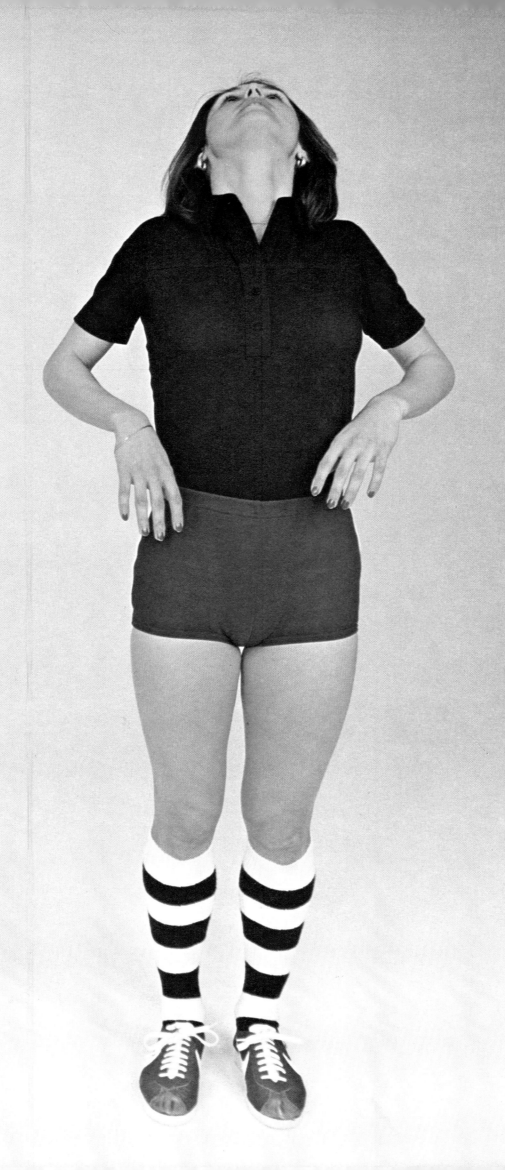

21 When performed in a smooth, rhythmical motion these side lunges look and feel good, as well as strengthening your thighs and abdominal muscles. The effort of each lunge is relieved by a downward body swing. In the lunge positions E and J your extended leg is bent at 90°—not more—with your toes pointed in the direction of the lunge. Your other leg is stretched straight with your toes pointed forward. Work on achieving a smooth transition between each change of position.

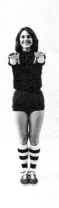

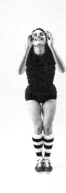

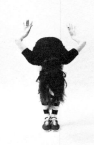

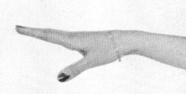

A Stand with your feet together and your arms forward at shoulder height.

B Swing down, bending your knees and relaxing your upper body.

C Finish the swing like this with your head coming down last.

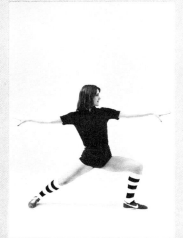

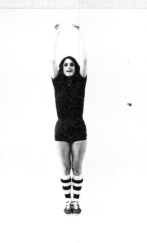

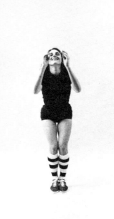

D Slowly straighten up, with your head coming up last.

E Lunge right by extending your right leg to your right side while stretching your arms to the sides.

F Move smoothly back to position **D**.

G Begin another downward swing as in **B**.

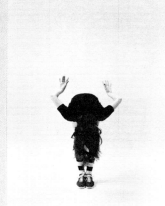

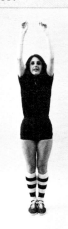

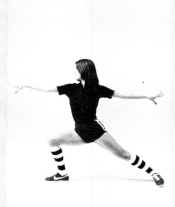

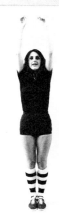

H Finish like this as in **C**.

I Straighten up to position **D**.

J Lunge left by extending your left leg to your left side while stretching your arms to the sides.

K Return smoothly to position **D** and repeat, beginning with **B**.

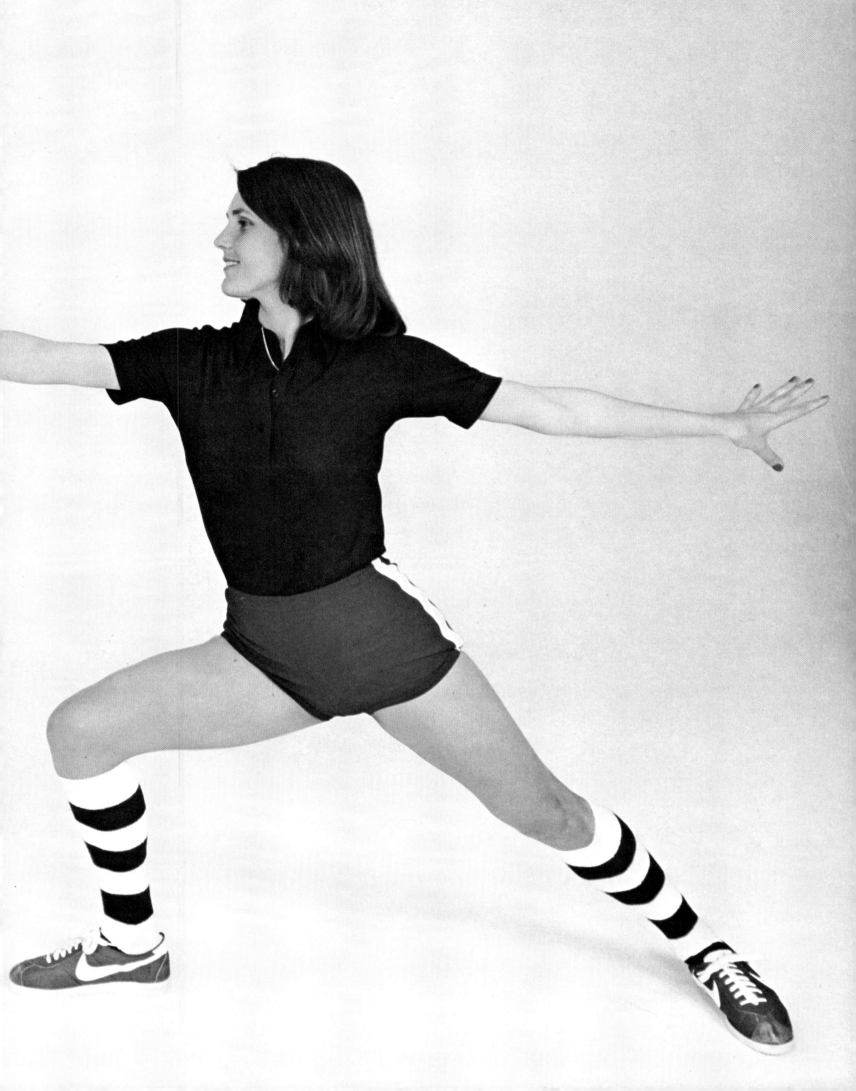

22 These stretches are beneficial to your upper back and arms, and slimming to your waistline. Pushing your arms to the sides and overhead strengthens your arms. Hold each position for a few seconds, making sure your shoulders are over your hips.

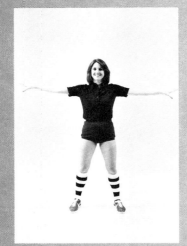

A Stand with your arms extended to the sides and feet shoulder width apart.

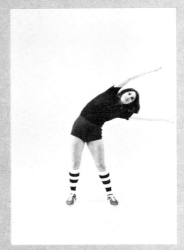

B Bend to the right bringing your left hand overhead like this.

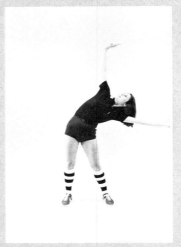

C Extend your left hand vertically and push up with your palm.

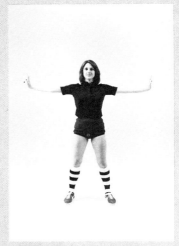

D Push both palms to the sides as if pushing against a wall.

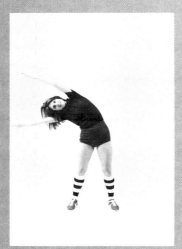

E Bend to the left bringing your right arm overhead like this.

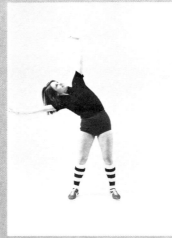

F Extend your right hand vertically and push up with your palm.

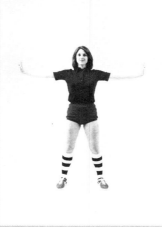

G Push both palms to the sides as in **D**. Repeat the sequence, beginning with **B**.

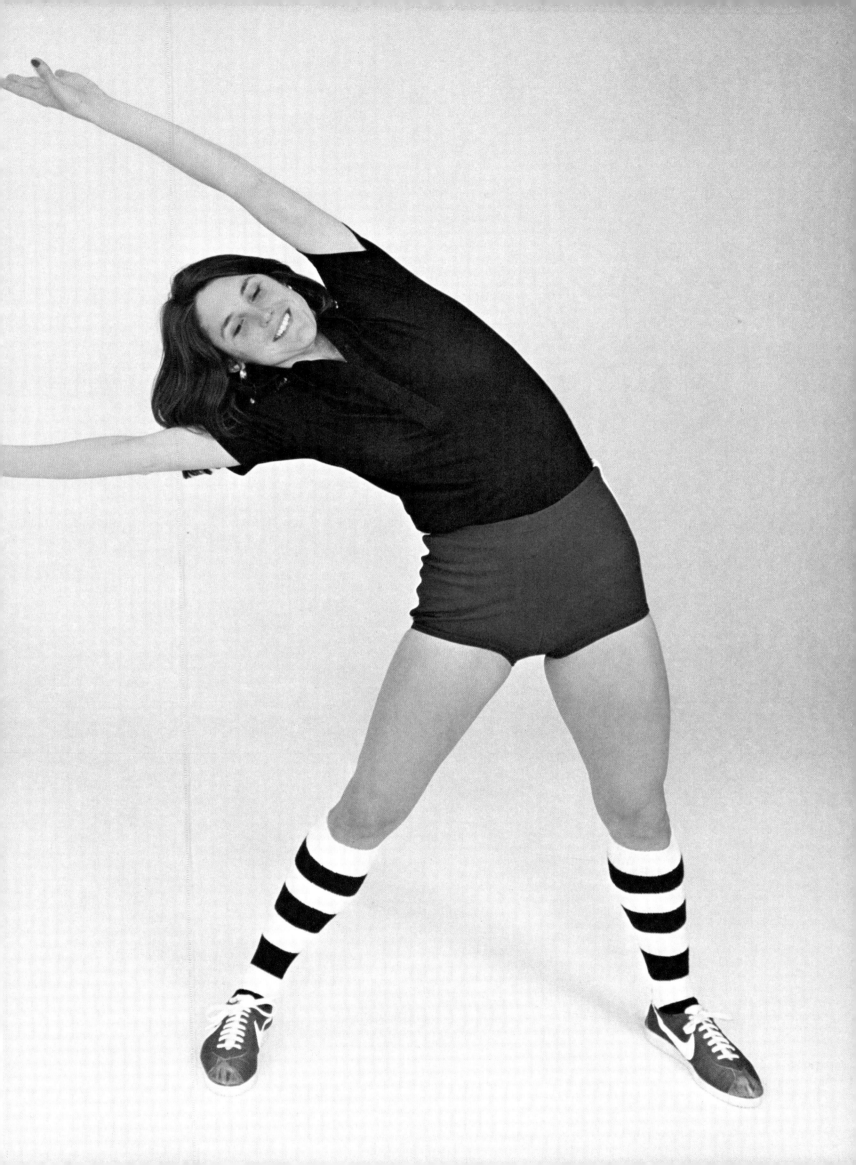

23

These overhead stretches help to slim your waistline while giving your shoulders, thighs and legs a workout. When stretching to each side avoid bending forward by keeping your shoulders in line with your hips.

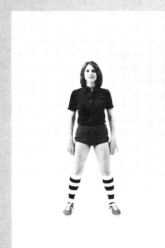

A Stand with your feet apart at shoulder width.

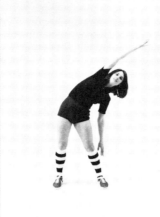

B Lean right, reaching your left arm overhead with the palm facing up.

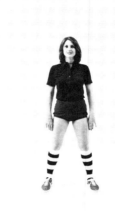

C Relax as in **A**.

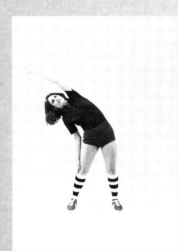

D Lean left, reaching your right arm overhead with the palm facing up.

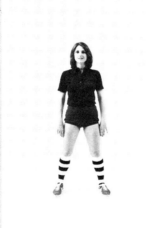

E. Relax.

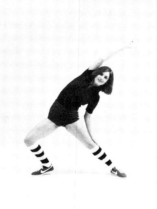

F Bending your left knee, lean right, reaching your left arm overhead with the palm facing up.

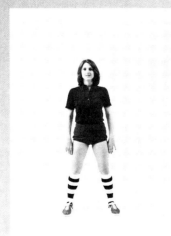

G Relax.

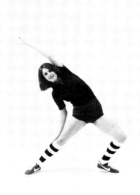

H Bending your right knee, lean left, reaching your right arm overhead with the palm facing up.

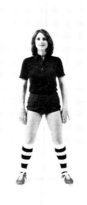

I Relax, then repeat, beginning with **B**.

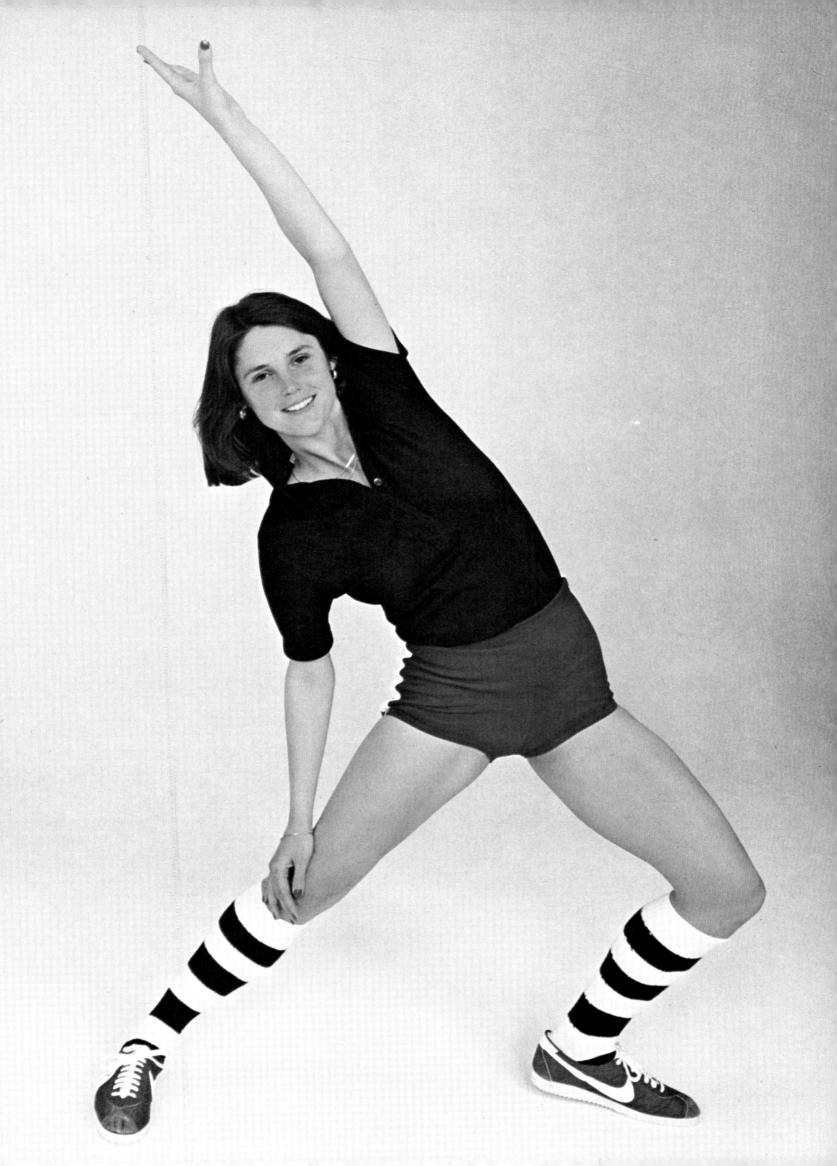

24 This Movement Pattern alternately stretches and strengthens your hamstring muscles and puts your balance and coordination to the test. Remember to fix your eye on a spot in front of you to maintain your balance, and concentrate on breathing evenly throughout. Try to keep your back straight as you extend your leg behind in E and J. When you reach up in E and J, don't reach behind but slightly in front. Perform the sequence slowly and smoothly.

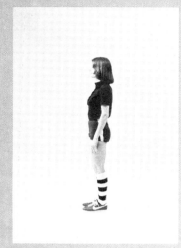

A Stand with your feet together.

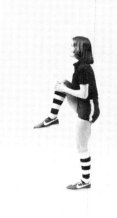

B Begin to raise your right knee and your arms.

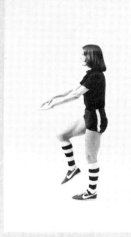

C Grasp your knee and pull it to your chest.

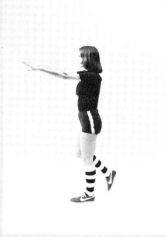

D Lower your right leg and extend it behind you while raising your arms.

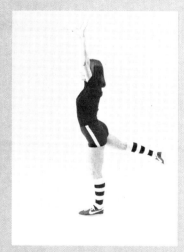

E Finish with your arms overhead and your leg extended behind with your knee locked.

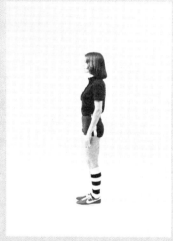

F Repeat the sequence **B** through **E** from four to twelve times, then return to **A**.

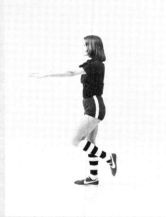

G Begin to raise your left knee and your arms.

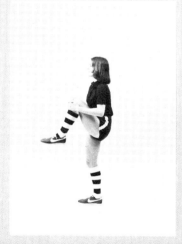

H Grasp your knee and pull it to your chest.

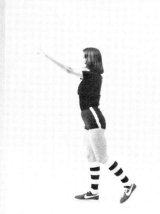

I Lower your left leg and extend it behind you while raising your arms.

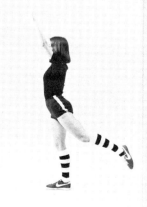

J Finish with your arms overhead and your leg extended behind with your knee locked.

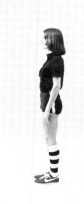

K Finish, after repeating the sequence **G** through **J** from four to twelve times.

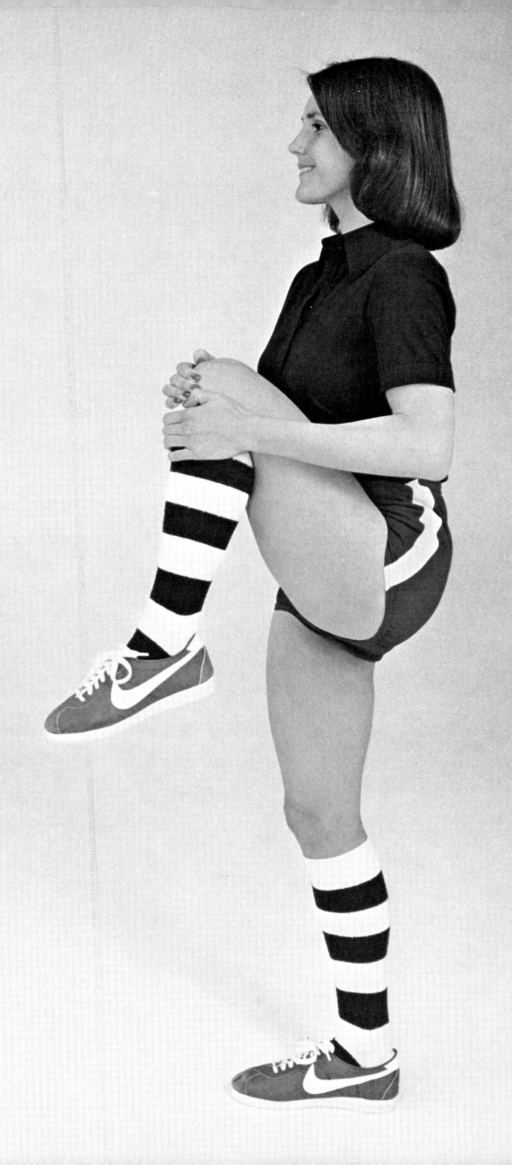

25 These waist circles stretch and slim your waistline. Use your hands to describe a wide circle around your body. Bend your knees as you bend at the waist, keeping them bent from C to F. Do the sequence shown in the photos twice, then do it twice in the opposite direction. Repeat the complete Movement Pattern from four to twelve times.

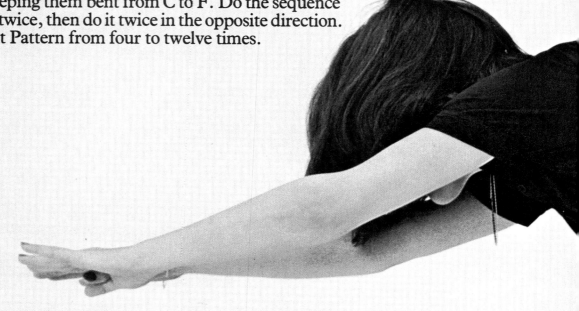

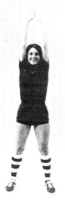

A Stand with your legs apart and your arms overhead with your thumbs interlocked.

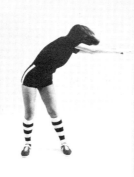

B Twist your upper body to face right.

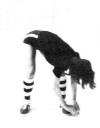

C Begin to swing down and bend your knees.

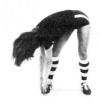

D Touch your right toe.

E Swing to the left and touch your left toe.

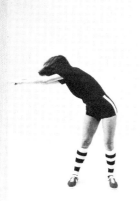

F Face left and swing upward, straightening your knees.

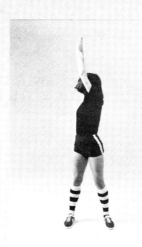

G Finish the swing with your arms overhead.

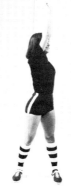

H Twist right and repeat, beginning with **B**.

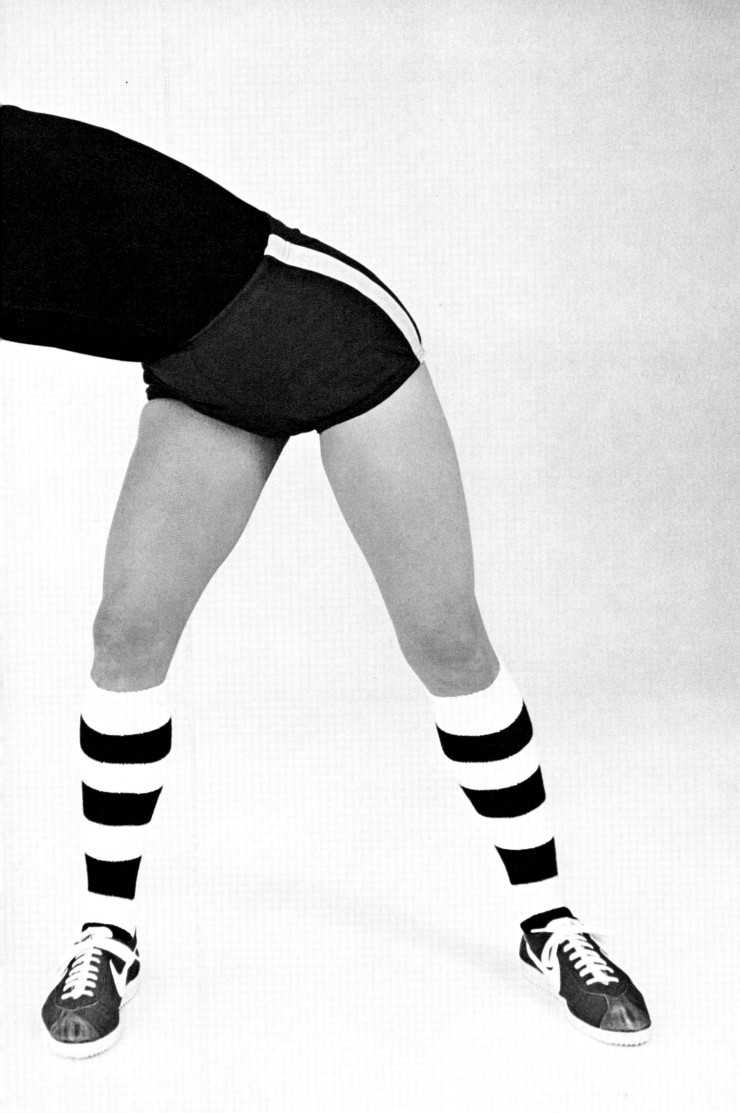

26 The next series of Movement Patterns is performed from a sitting or lying position. This one stretches your hamstring muscles and increases the strength of your abdominal muscles. When rolling backward and forward keep your head as close as possible to your knee. Your abdominal muscles control the rolling action, which should be done at a smooth and even pace without jerking or bouncing. Your knees may bend slightly.

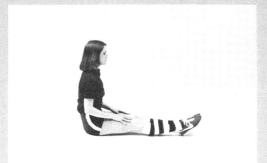

A Sit with your legs together in front of you.

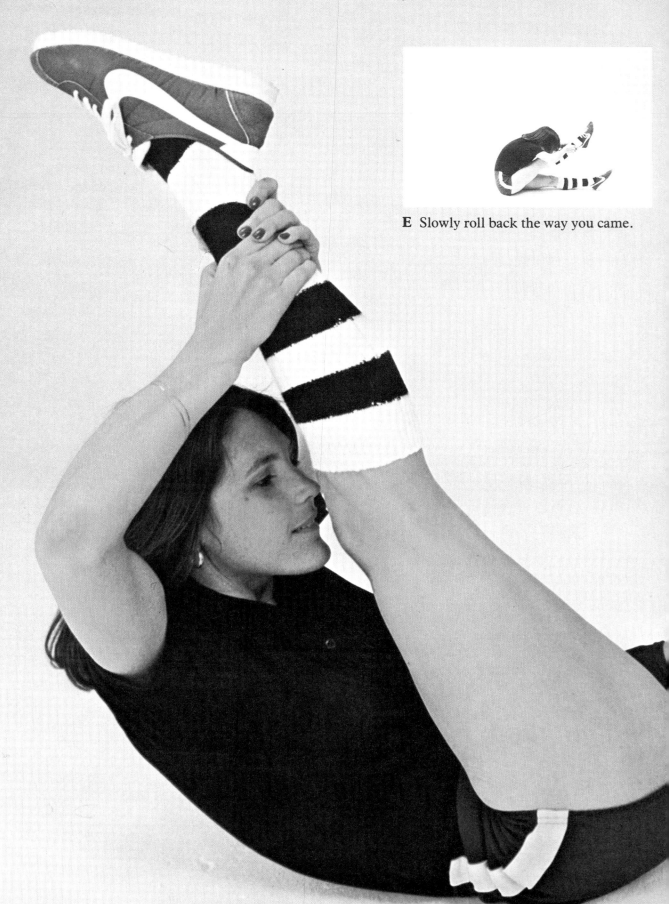

E Slowly roll back the way you came.

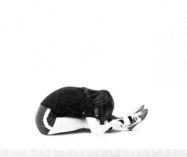

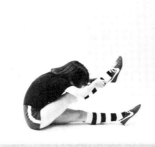

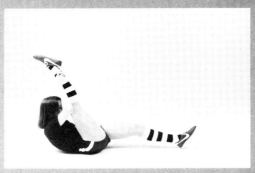

B Reach forward and grasp your right ankle.

C Slowly roll backward, pulling your leg to your chest and contracting your abdominal muscles.

D Finish like this, pressing the small of your back to the floor.

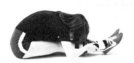

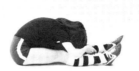

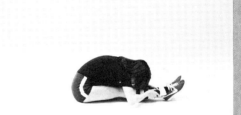

F Finish as you started in **B.**

G Grasp your left ankle.

H Slowly roll backward, pulling your leg to your chest and contracting your abdominal muscles.

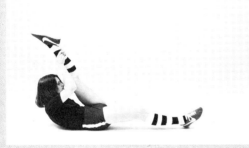

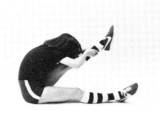

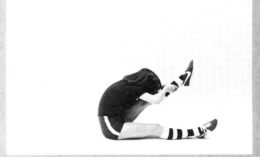

I Finish like this, pressing the small of your back to the floor.

J Slowly roll back the way you came.

K Finish by grasping your right ankle and repeat, beginning with **C.**

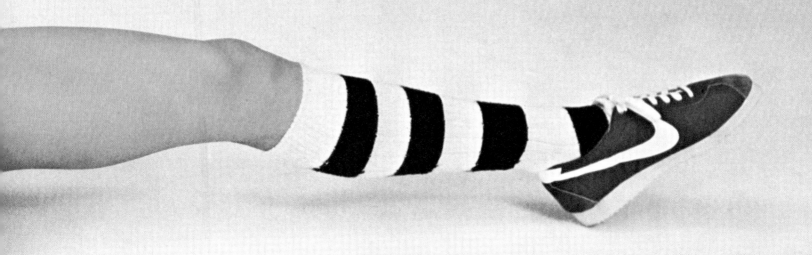

27 These back rolls strengthen your abdominal muscles and stretch your lower back and hamstring muscles. Work on developing a fluid and even transition between each phase of movement. Make sure your knees are bent when you're rolling backward or forward. In E, F and G keep your head moving forward; this aids in curling your spine and helps to prevent you from arching your back. In H and I keep your chin tucked to your chest until your shoulders touch the floor.

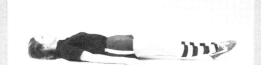
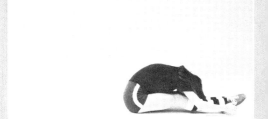

A Lie with your legs together, your arms at your sides with your palms facing down, and push the small of your back to the floor.

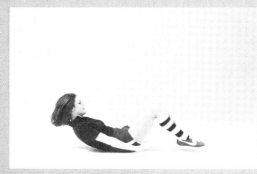

E Extend your legs forward and roll up with your upper body.

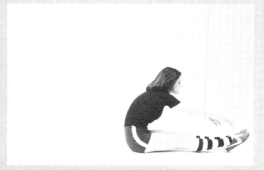

F Continue to roll forward, reaching for your ankles.

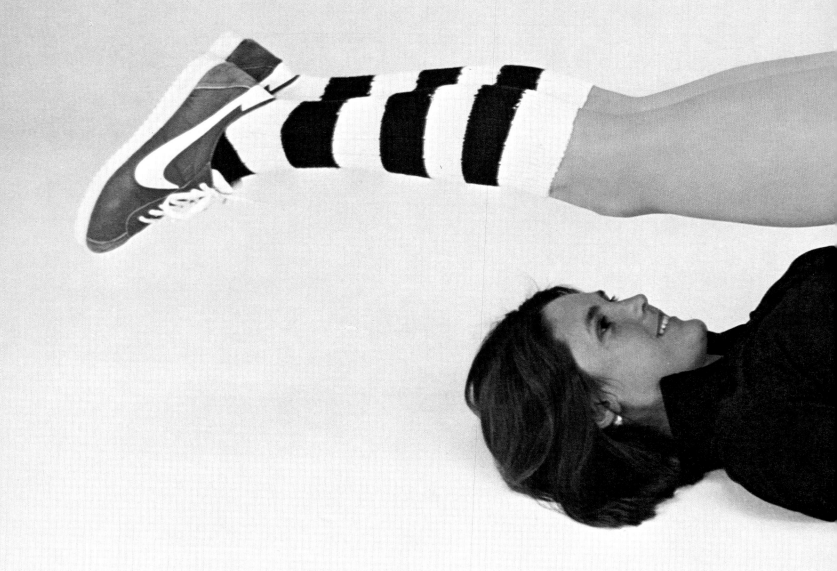

G Grasp your ankles and gently pull your chest toward your thighs.

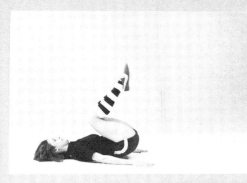

B Tuck your knees to your chest.

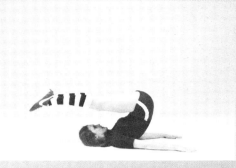

C Lift your hips and extend your legs over your head, parallel to the floor.

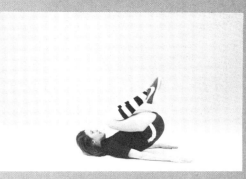

D Bend your knees back into a tuck position.

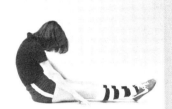

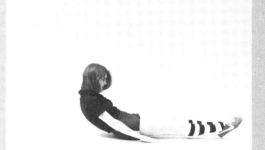

H Slowly roll back from **G**, touching your chin to your chest.

I Roll back to the floor.

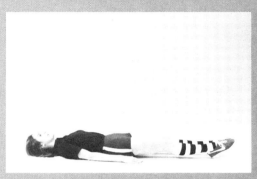

J Resume position **A** and repeat, beginning with **B.**

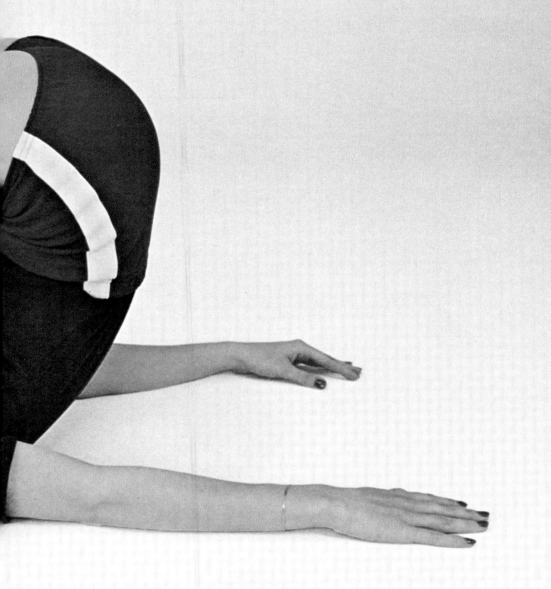

28 These sit ups are a progression from the back roll series in 27. They are particularly good for developing your abdominal strength and stretching your hamstrings. Again you should perform the sequence in one continuous fluid motion. Let your abdominal muscles control your movement. In B and C bring your upper body and knees together in a jacknife motion. Slide your hands along your body in G and H to assist you in keeping your head tucked and your spine curled.

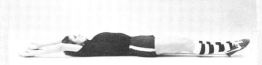

A Lie with your legs together and your arms stretched overhead.

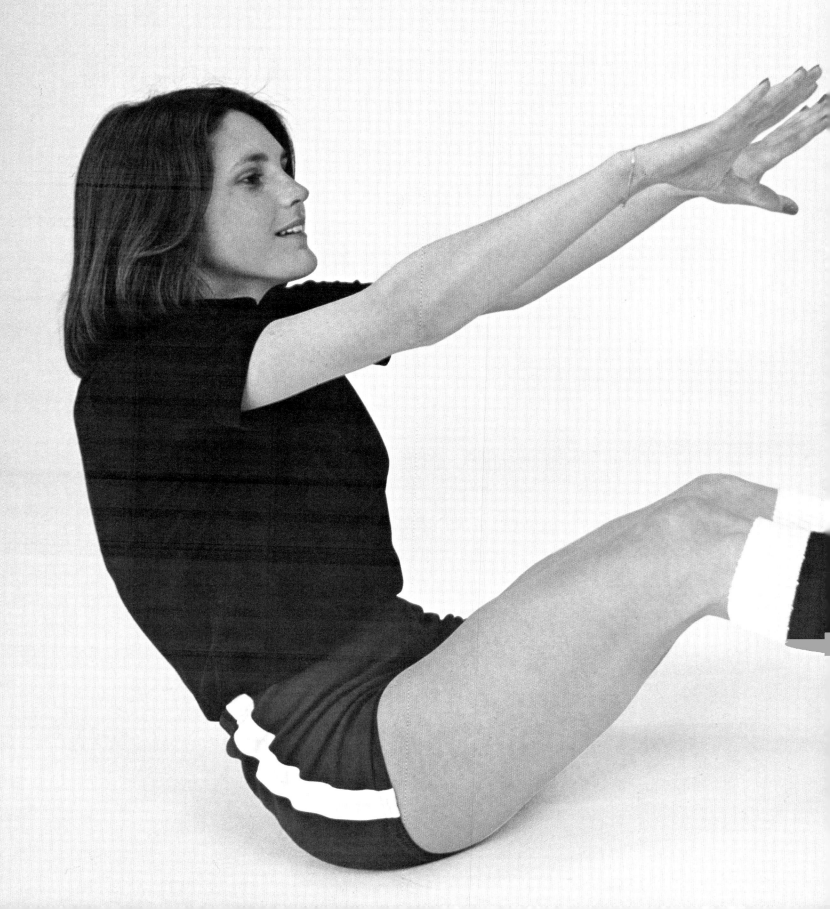

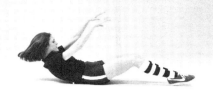

B Raise your upper body and knees together.

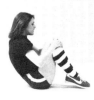

C Sit up to this position with your back rounded and grasp your knees.

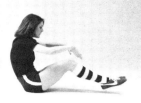

D Release your knees and lower them.

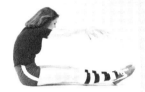

E Extend your legs and lean forward.

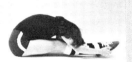

F Finish like this by grasping your ankles and pulling yourself over your thighs.

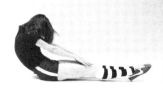

G Release your ankles and begin to roll back the way you came.

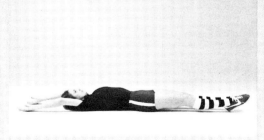

H Continue to roll back smoothly with your chin tucked to your chest.

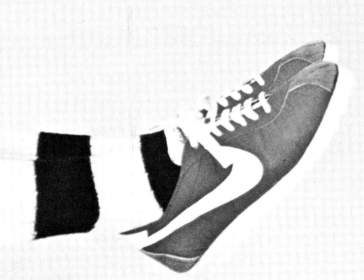

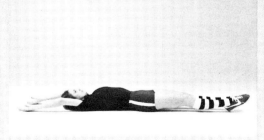

I Finish as in **A**, with your head coming down last. Repeat, beginning with **B**.

29 Your back, thigh and abdominal muscles are strengthened by this Movement Pattern. You may lean forward slightly in this sequence but avoid leaning back, particularly in E and I. Round your back as you pull your knee to your chest.

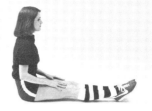

A Sit with your legs together in front of you.

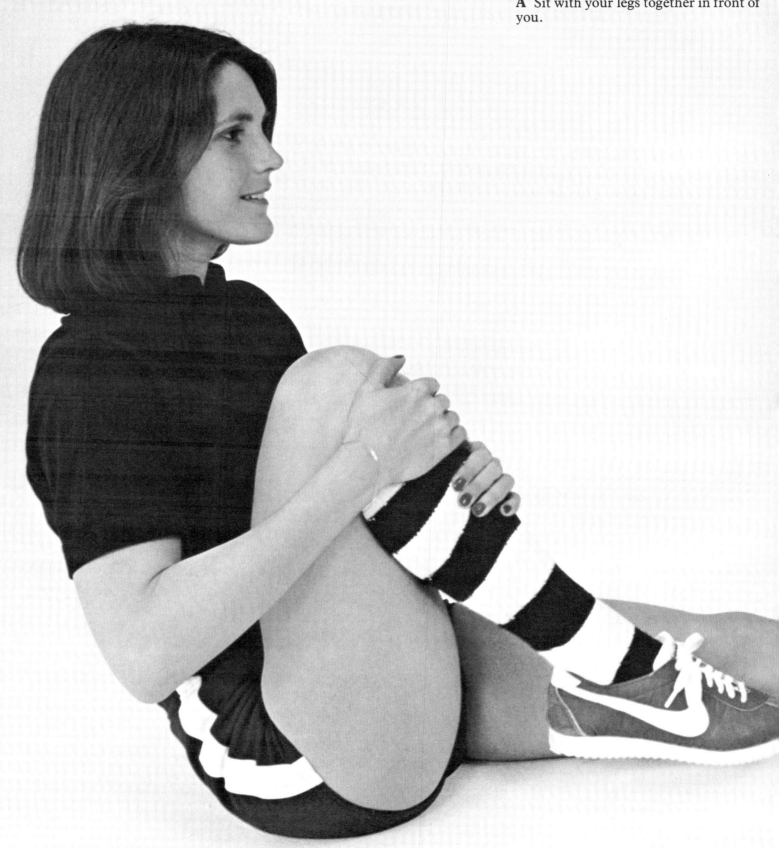

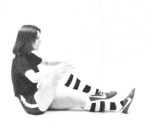 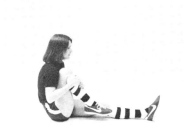 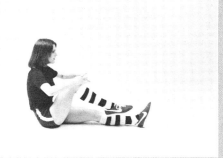

B Reach for your right knee as you raise it.

C Pull your right knee to your chest.

D Return your leg to the floor.

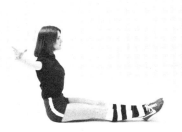 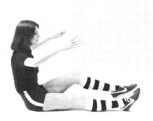 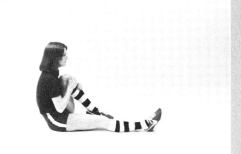

E Reach to the sides.

F Reach for your left knee as you raise it.

G Pull your left knee to your chest.

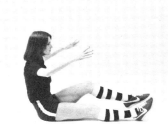

H Return your leg to the floor.

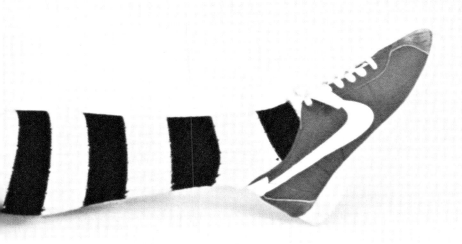

I Reach to the sides, then repeat beginning with **B**.

30 This sequence relieves the tension in your abdominal muscles after the concentration placed on them in the previous Movement Patterns. The muscles in your arms, back, hips, buttocks and legs are all used as well. When raising your body in F tuck your chin to your chest, look at your toes, and try to place your body in a straight line from your heels to your shoulders.

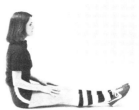

A Sit with your legs together in front of you.

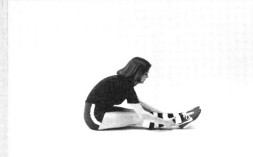

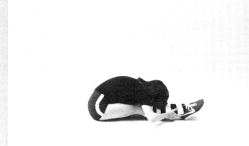

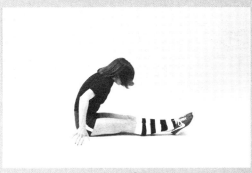

B Grasp your ankles and pull your chest toward your thighs.

C Finish like this.

D Uncurl the way you came.

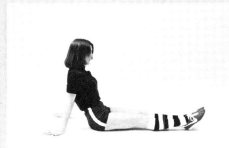

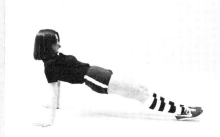

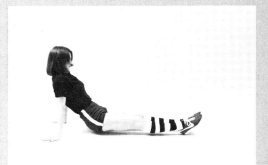

E Place your hands behind your hips.

F Raise your body from the floor, pinching your buttocks together and pushing your hips toward the ceiling.

G Lower to the floor then repeat, beginning with **B**.

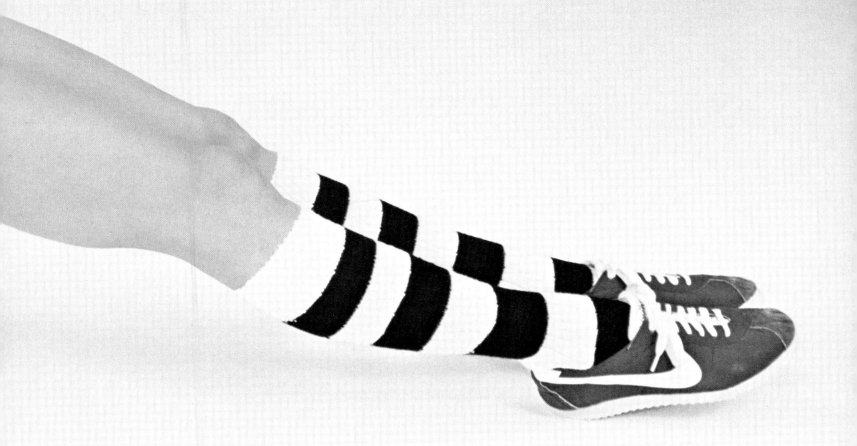

31

Rotating your hips and thighs in this way improves the flexibility of your hips, strengthens your thighs and firms your buttocks. It also helps to slim your waistline. Follow the movement of your leg with your eyes.

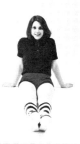

A Sit with your legs in front and your hands on the floor behind you.

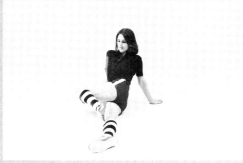

C Rotate your right knee over to the floor on your left side.

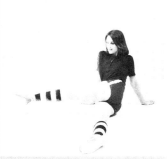

D Straighten your right leg.

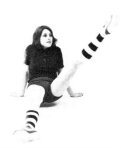

E Raise your right leg straight up and over to your right side.

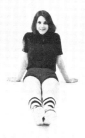

G Resume position **A**.

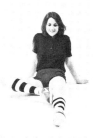

H Place your left foot on your right knee.

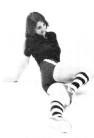

I Rotate your left knee over to the floor on your right side.

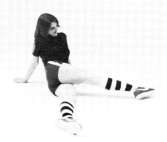

J Straighten your left leg.

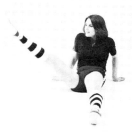

K Raise your left leg straight up and over to your left side.

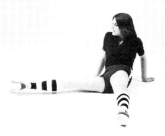

L Lower your leg to finish like this, then begin again with **B**.

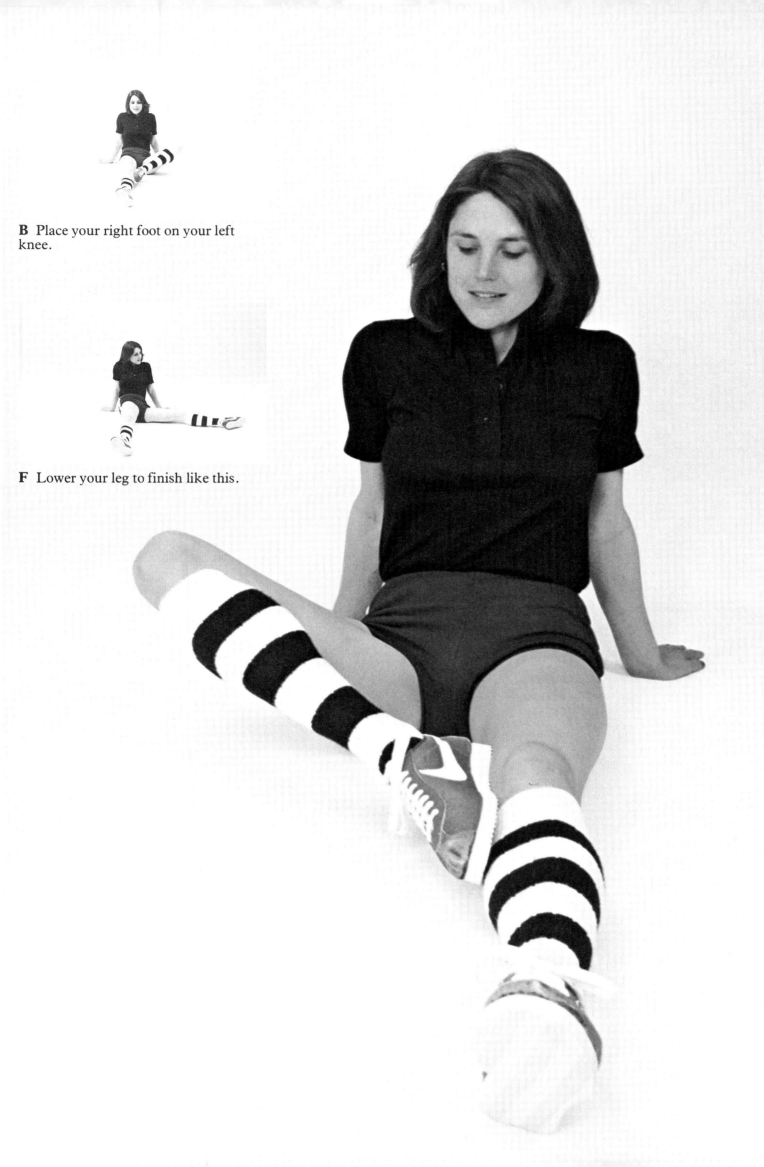

B Place your right foot on your left knee.

F Lower your leg to finish like this.

32 Sitting up this way, with your knees raised, strengthens your neck and upper abdominal muscles while relieving any tension in your lower back. As a bonus it also helps to slim your waistline when you twist in the second half of the Movement Pattern. Perform this sequence slowly, smoothly and rhythmically. Touch your forehead to your knees in B and D if you can.

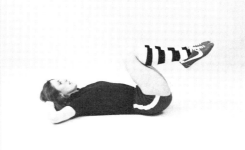

A Lie with your knees bent, your feet off the floor and your hands clasped behind your head.

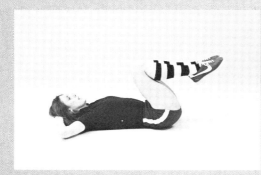

E Slowly uncurl again as in **C**.

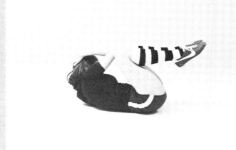

F Curl up and twist at your waist to touch your right elbow to your left knee.

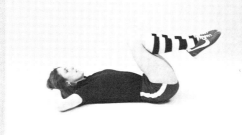

G Uncurl back to **E**.

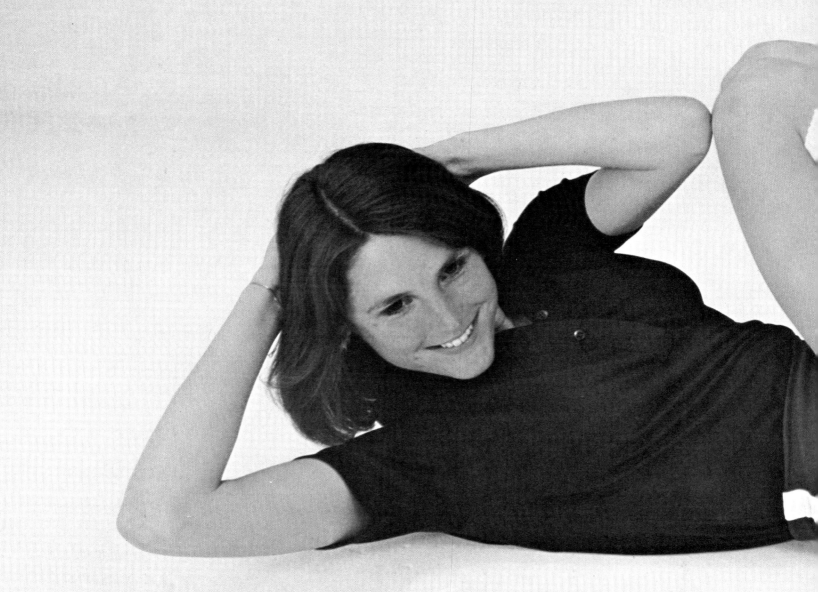

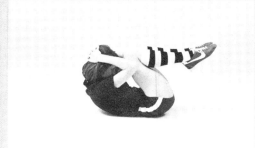

B Curl up toward your knees.

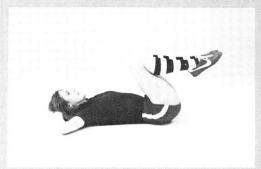

C Slowly uncurl back to **A.**

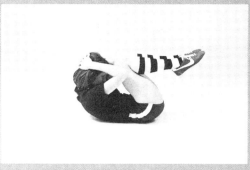

D Curl up toward your knees again.

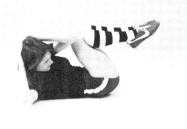

H Curl up and twist at your waist to touch your left elbow to your right knee.

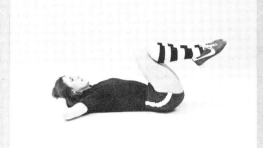

I Uncurl back to the floor and repeat, beginning with **B.**

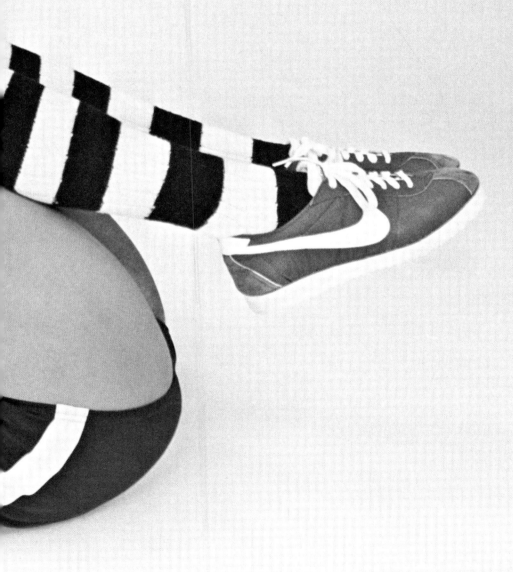

33 The next series of Movement Patterns is performed from a reclining position. This first exercise stretches your hamstrings, gives your neck muscles a workout and relieves tension in your back. When raising your head and shoulders in F and H keep your lower back on the floor. Touch your nose to your knee if you can.

A Lie with your legs together and your arms extended overhead.

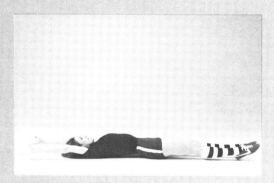

E Return your leg to the floor.

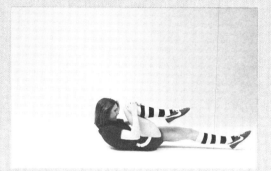

F Pull your right knee toward your chest and raise your nose toward it.

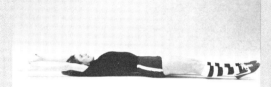

G Lower to the floor.

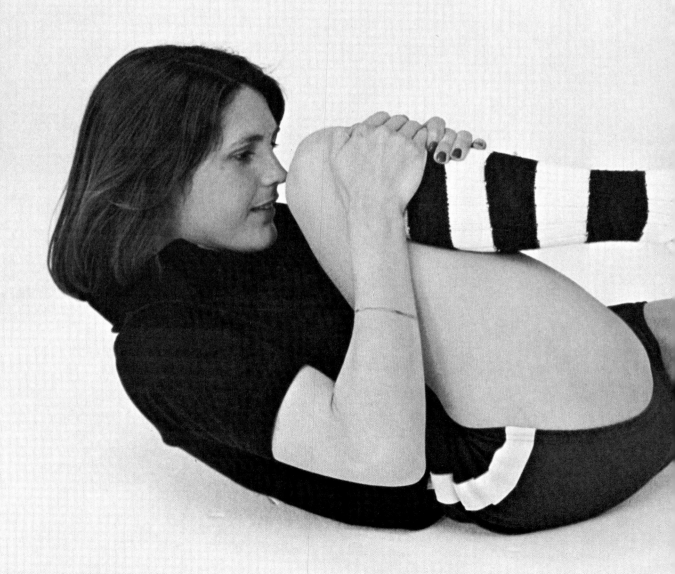

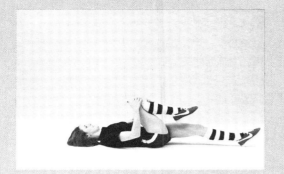

B Pull your right knee toward your chest.

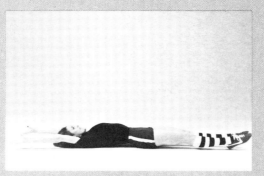

C Return your leg to the floor.

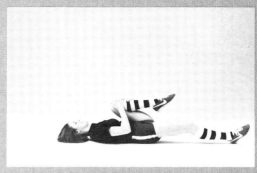

D Pull your left knee toward your chest.

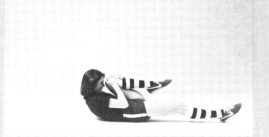

H Pull your left knee toward your chest and raise your nose toward it.

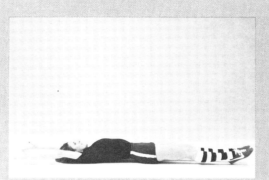

I Lower to the floor and repeat, beginning with **B**.

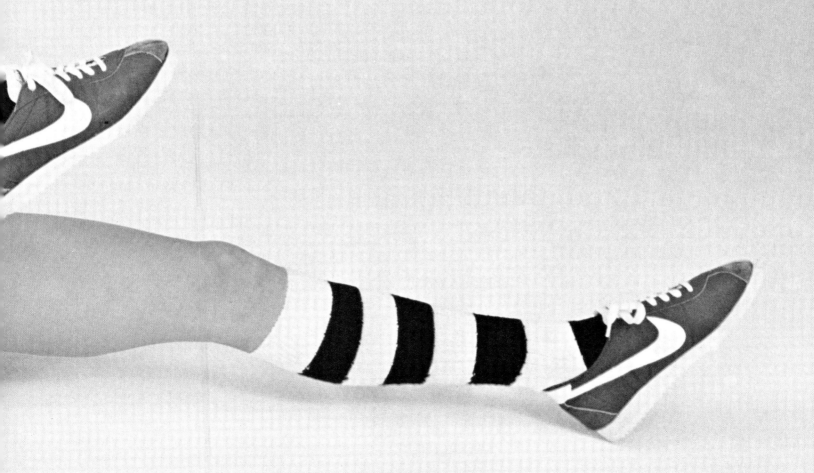

34 Your hips and thighs are strengthened and firmed by these leg crossovers. Your waist is stretched as your leg is lowered to the sides. Raise and lower your leg slowly in each case, avoiding a sudden movement. Control the speed with your abdominal and thigh muscles. Press the small of your back to the floor as you raise your leg. Your arms might lift slightly from the floor as you lower your leg in C and H.

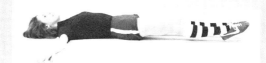

A Lie with your legs together and your arms extended to each side.

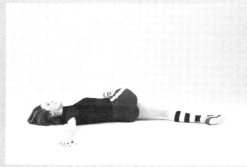

D Finish with your foot touching the floor.

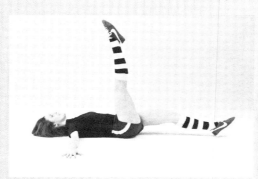

E Return your leg to the vertical position.

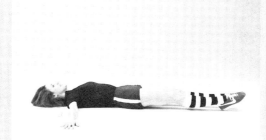

F Lower your leg.

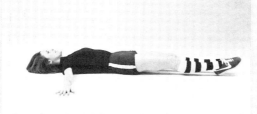

I Finish with your foot touching the floor.

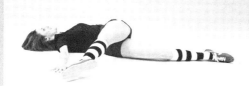

K Lower your leg and repeat, beginning with **B.**

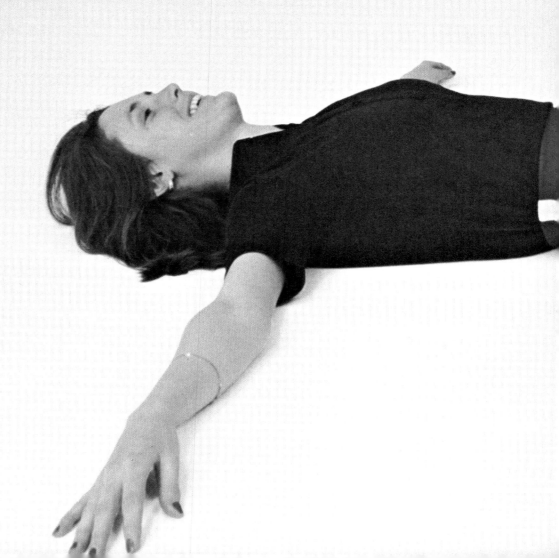

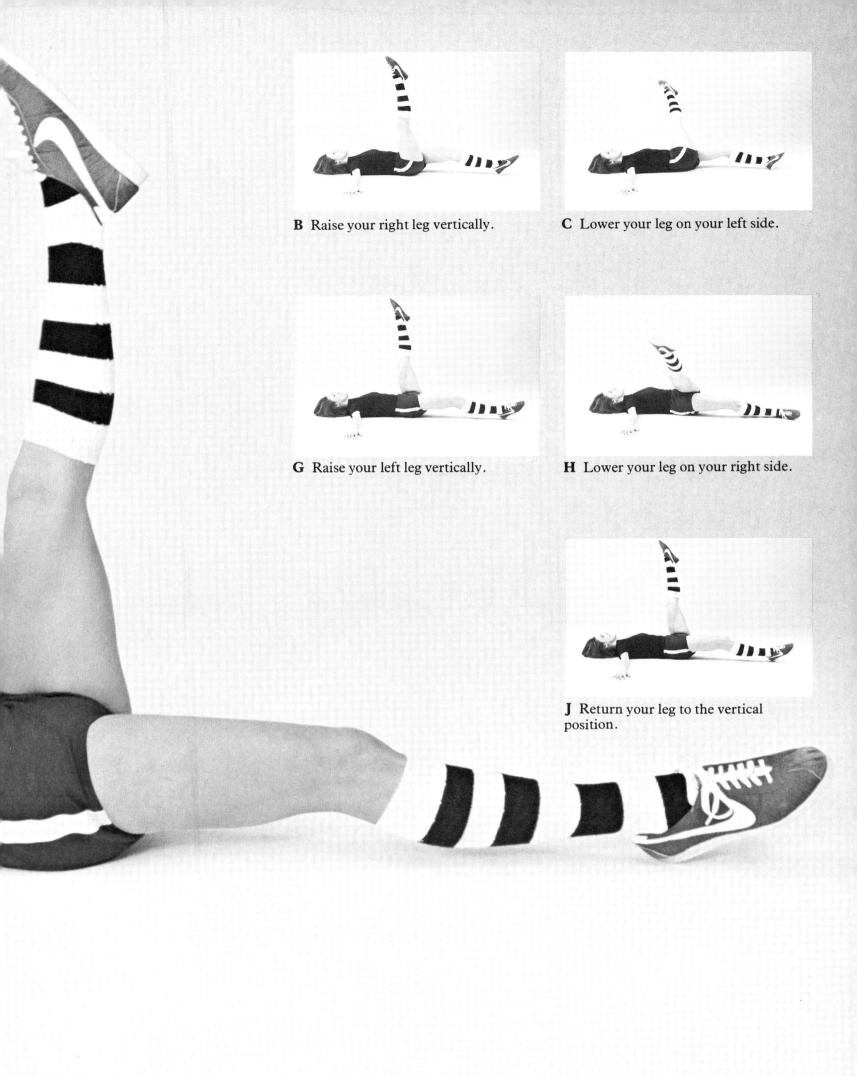

B Raise your right leg vertically.

C Lower your leg on your left side.

G Raise your left leg vertically.

H Lower your leg on your right side.

J Return your leg to the vertical position.

35 This Movement Pattern stretches your abdominal and hip muscles and strengthens your thighs. In E and H your body should be in a straight line. You can achieve this by sighting along your leg to check that it's in line with your upper body.

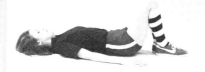

A Lie with your legs together, your knees bent and your arms at your sides.

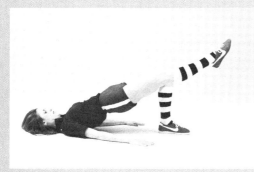

E Raise your right leg and your hips simultaneously.

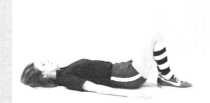

F Lower your hips and leg while bending your knee. Finish like this, as in **C**.

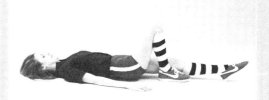

G Extend your left leg.

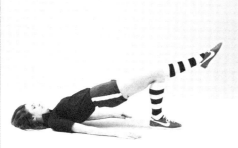

H Raise your left leg and your hips simultaneously.

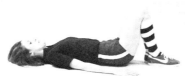

I Lower your hips and leg while bending your knee as in **F**. Finish like this then repeat, beginning with **B**.

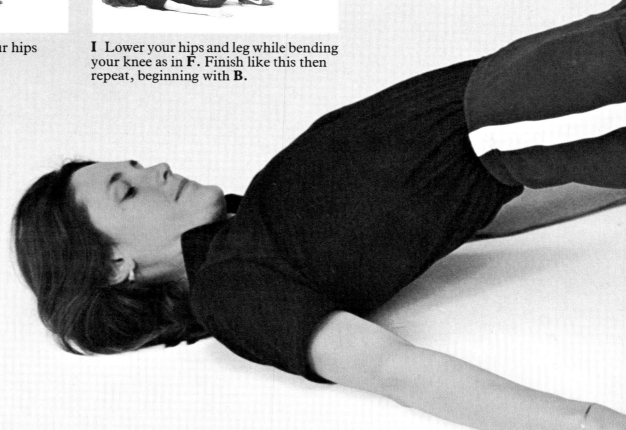

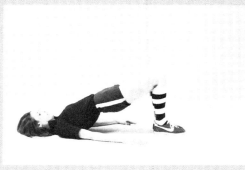

B Raise your hips.

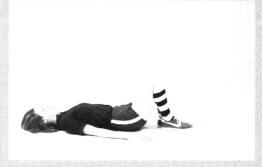

C Lower your hips.

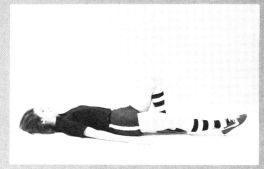

D Extend your right leg.

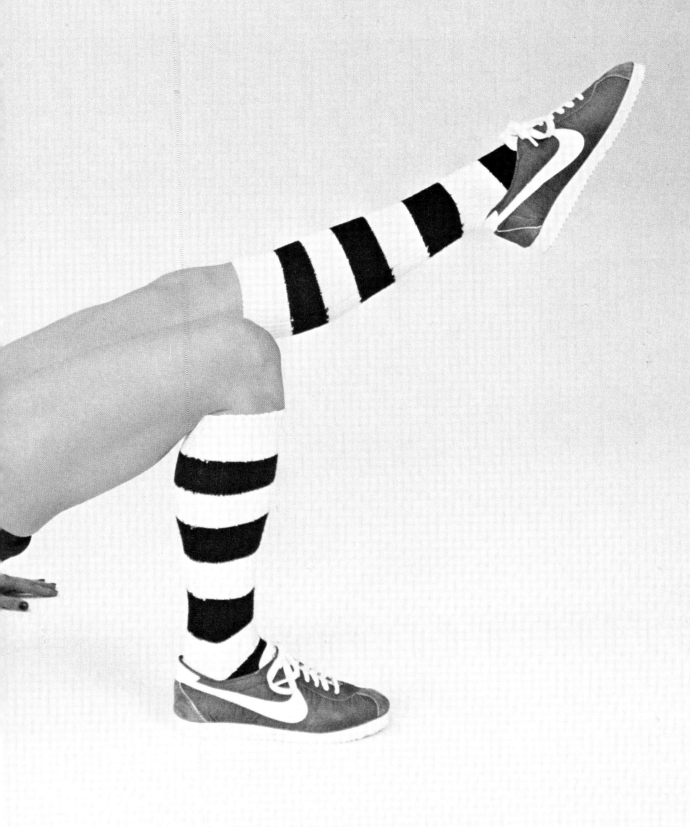

36 The trick in this Movement Pattern, which strengthens your abdomen and the muscles in the front of your thighs, is to raise and lower your opposite arm and leg simultaneously. Practice doing this in a smooth motion. Press the small of your back to the floor in A, D and G.

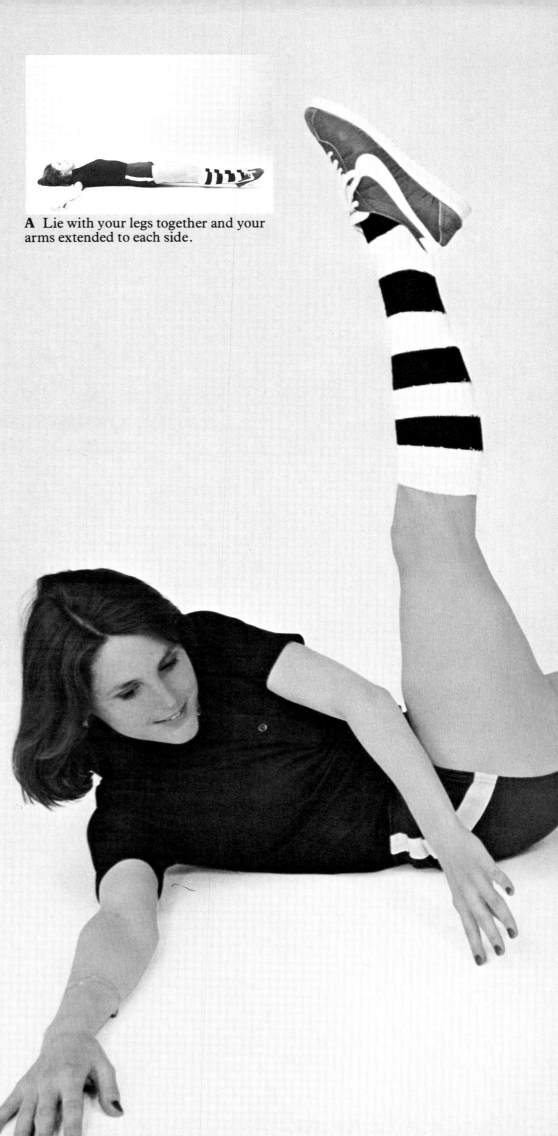

A Lie with your legs together and your arms extended to each side.

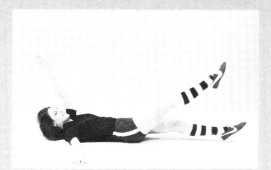

B Raise your right leg and left arm while lifting your left shoulder.

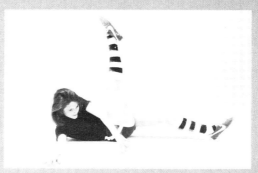

C Finish with your right leg vertical and your left arm across your body touching the floor.

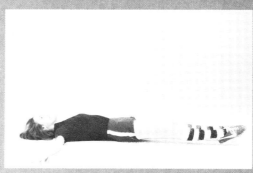

D Slowly lower to the floor as in **A**.

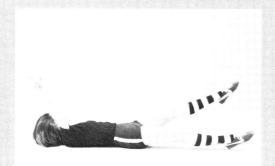

E Raise your left leg and right arm while lifting your right shoulder.

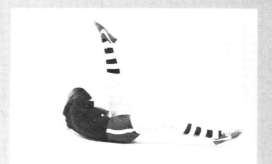

F Finish with your left leg vertical and your right arm across your body touching the floor.

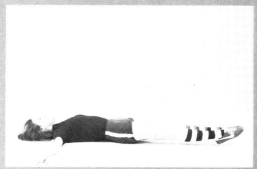

G Slowly lower to the floor then repeat, beginning with **B**.

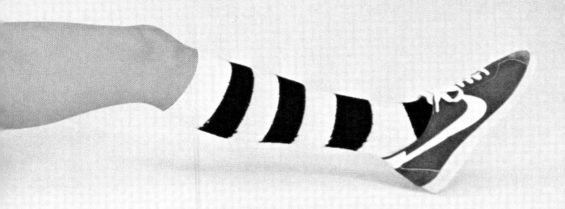

37

Swinging your legs in an arc from side to side in this way increases your thigh and abdominal muscle strength as well as improving the flexibility of your hips. Throughout this sequence press your arms and back against the floor to assist you in keeping your leg in the air without arching your back. Point your toe in the direction of your leg movement to help rotate your hips. Your hips may roll when your leg crosses over in C and G. Swing your leg in an arc, low in the middle and high on the sides. Perform each arc four times.

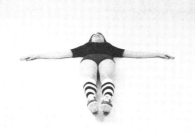

A Lie with your arms extended to the sides and your legs together.

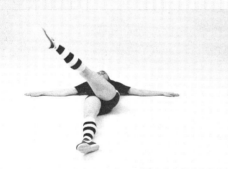

B Raise your right leg high to your right side.

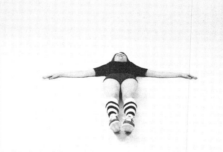

C Swing it to your left in an arc, low in the centre.

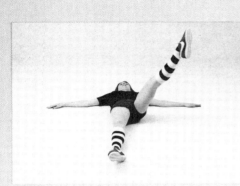

D Finish the arc high over your left side. Swing from **B** to **D** four times.

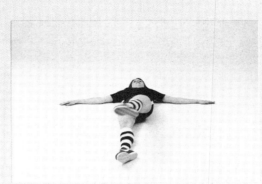

E Return your leg to the floor.

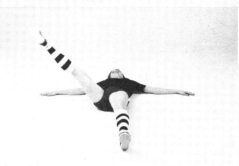

F Raise your left leg high to your left side.

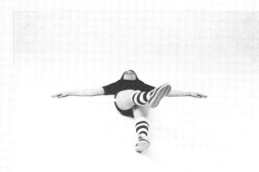

G Swing it to your right in an arc, low in the centre.

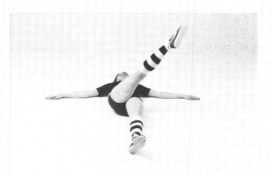

H Finish the arc high over your right side. Swing from **F** to **H** four times.

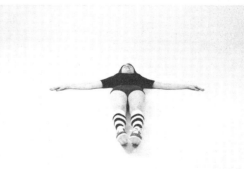

I Return to **A**, then begin again with **B**.

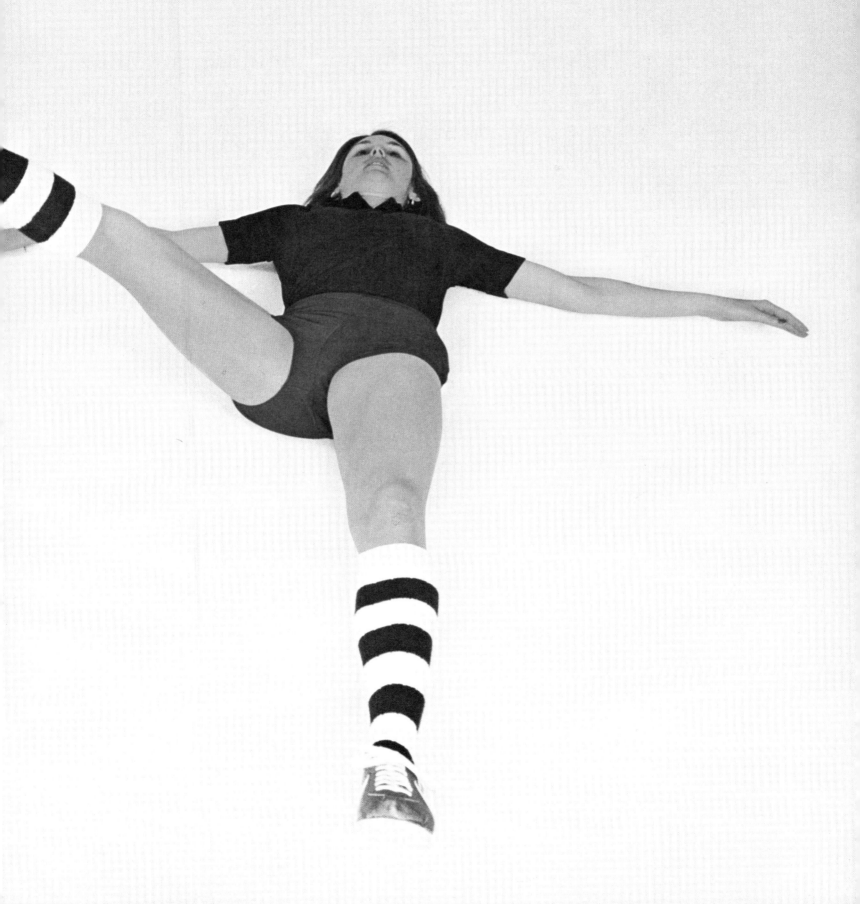

38

This Movement Pattern is similar to the previous one, but your legs now describe a figure 8 pattern in the air instead of an arc. Once again you should keep your arms and the small of your back pressed to the floor, and point your toe in the direction of your leg movement. Your hips may roll when your leg crosses over in D and I. To perform the figure 8 (actually an 8 on its side) imagine that you are drawing an 8 with your toe. Draw one half of the 8 on each side.

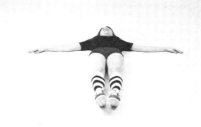

A Lie with your arms extended to the sides and your legs together.

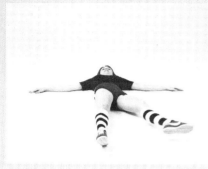

B Begin a circle to your right with your right leg.

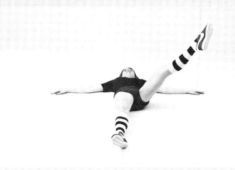

C Make a wide and high circle.

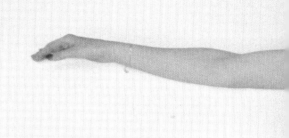

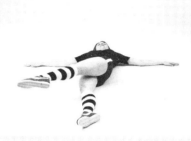

D Lower your leg to finish the circle and then cross it over to your left side.

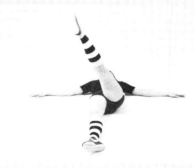

E Raise your leg in another wide and high circle to your left.

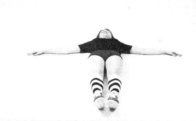

F Lower your leg to finish the figure 8.

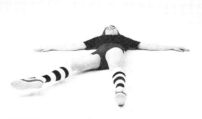

G Begin a circle to your left with your left leg.

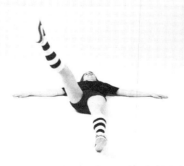

H Make a wide and high circle.

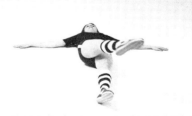

I Lower your leg to finish the circle and then cross it over to your right side.

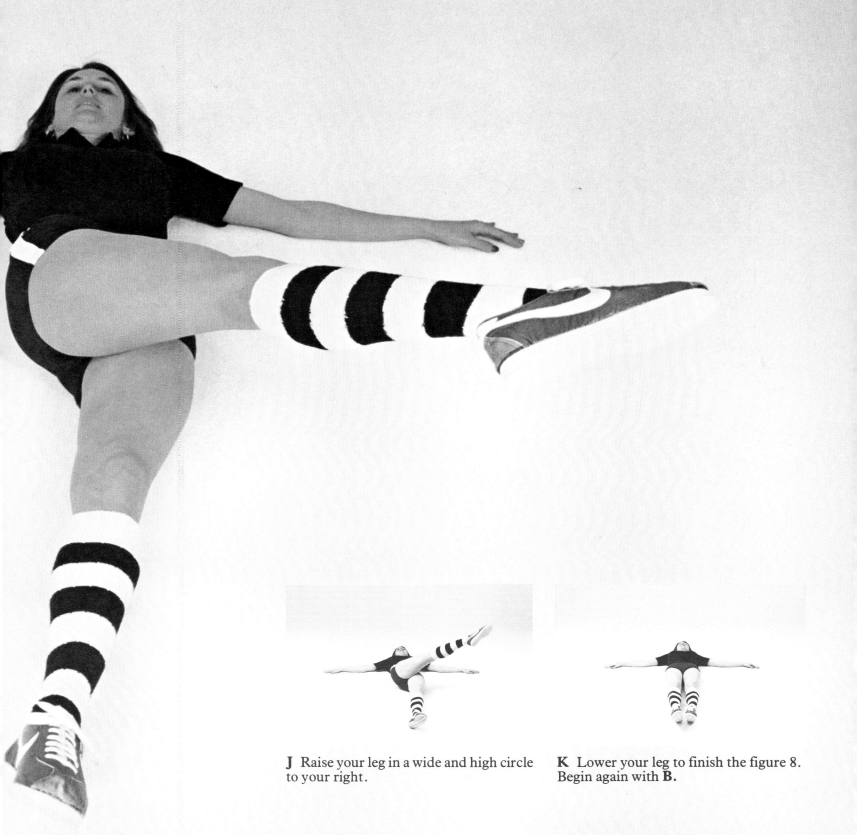

J Raise your leg in a wide and high circle to your right.

K Lower your leg to finish the figure 8. Begin again with **B.**

39 Sit ups with accompanying arm circles increase your abdominal strength and improve the flexibility of your shoulders. Combine the stages of this sequence into one fluid motion. Your feet should remain on the floor throughout the sequence. Your arms describe a complete circle from **B** through **F**. This provides momentum to assist you in raising your upper body to your knees and helps you to keep your spine rounded as you sit up.

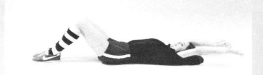

A Lie with your knees bent and your arms stretched overhead.

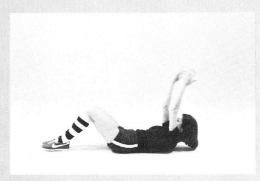

B Begin to circle your arms forward and curl upward with your head and shoulders.

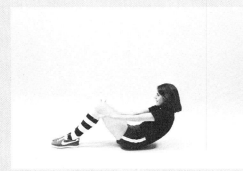

C Follow your arms to your knees.

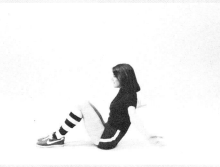

D Continue your arms in a circle down and behind you as you continue to come forward.

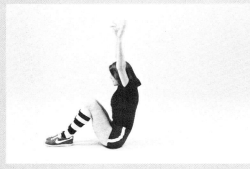

E Bring your arms up and overhead, as your chest approaches your knees.

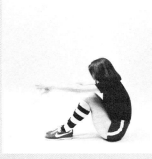

F Stretch your arms in front and round your back over your knees.

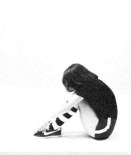

G Touch your toes, bending over your knees with your head down.

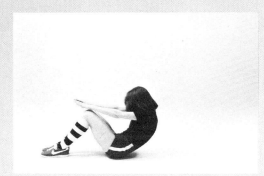

I Touch your knees as you continue back and down.

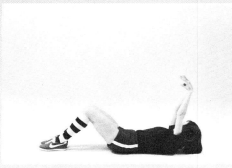

J Return to the floor with your arms following overhead.

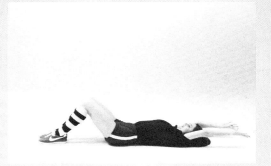

K Resume position **A** and repeat, beginning with **B**.

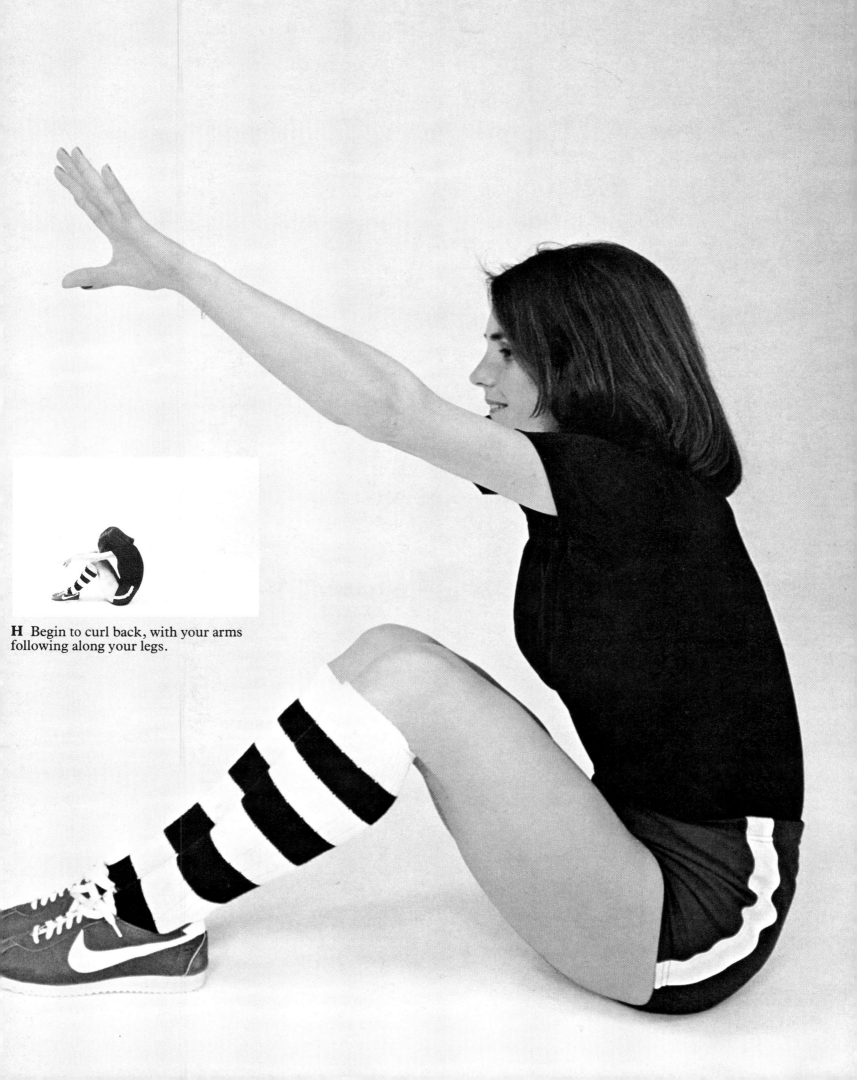

H Begin to curl back, with your arms following along your legs.

40 One of the benefits of this Movement Pattern is the relief of lower back pain. When you stretch your hamstrings their pull on your lower back is reduced. Your hip and thigh muscles are also strengthened. Stretch only as far as comfortable and keep your back as flat as possible. Your knees may bend slightly as you stretch forward. In F keep your chin tucked to your chest and your body in a straight line. Avoid arching your back.

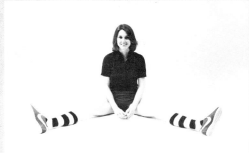

A Sit with your legs wide apart.

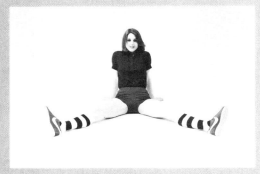

E Uncurl to a sitting position, with your hands on the floor behind your hips.

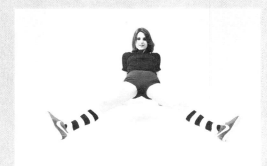

F Raise your hips off the floor.

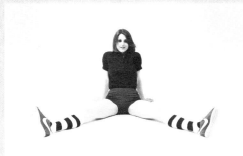

G Lower to the floor then repeat, beginning with **B.**

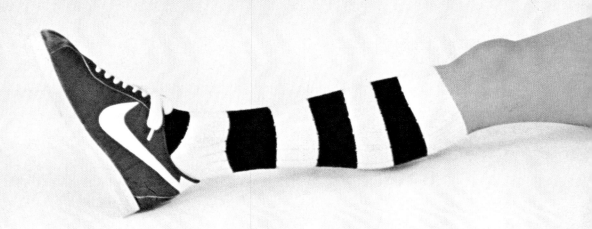

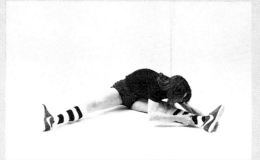 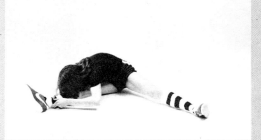 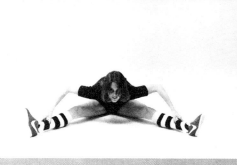

B Grasp your right ankle and try to place your ribs on your right thigh.

C Grasp your left ankle and try to place your ribs on your left thigh.

D Grasp both ankles and press your chest toward the floor.

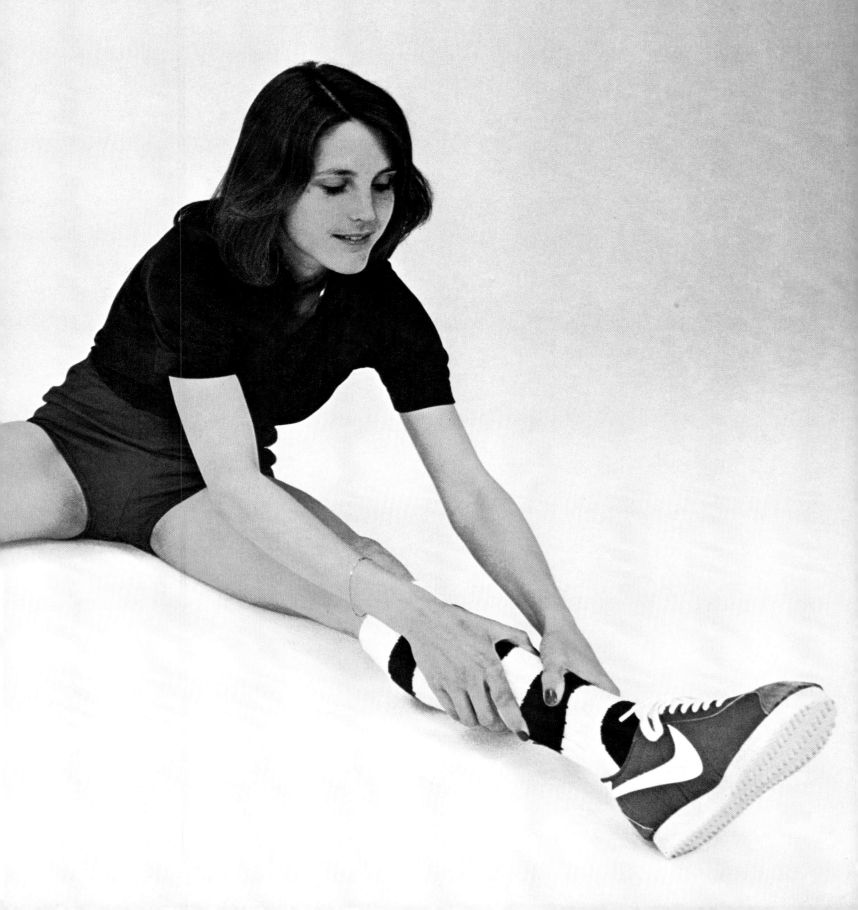

41 These leg exchanges, which strengthen your arms, legs and abdomen, are accompanied by a 'bouncing' movement. This is accomplished by raising and lowering your hips close to the floor–without touching it–at a rhythmical pace throughout the sequence. Lower your hips as you extend your leg in B and D, and raise them in C. Concentrate on placing your heels on the floor gently. Exchange your legs at a comfortable speed and continue this Movement Pattern for at least one minute.

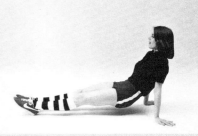

A Sit with your weight on your hands and heels and your hips off the floor and begin to bounce lightly.

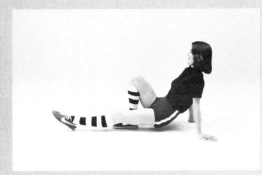

B Bring your right foot to your hips.

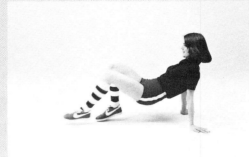

C Exchange legs.

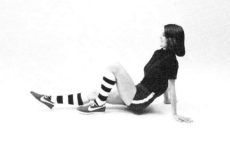

D Finish like this with your left foot at your hips. Continue exchanging legs.

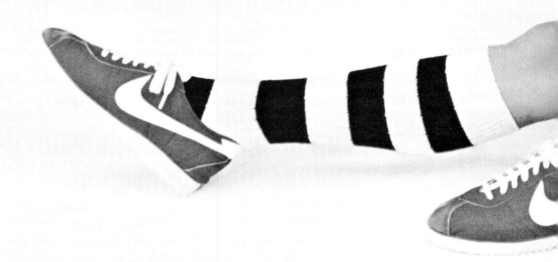

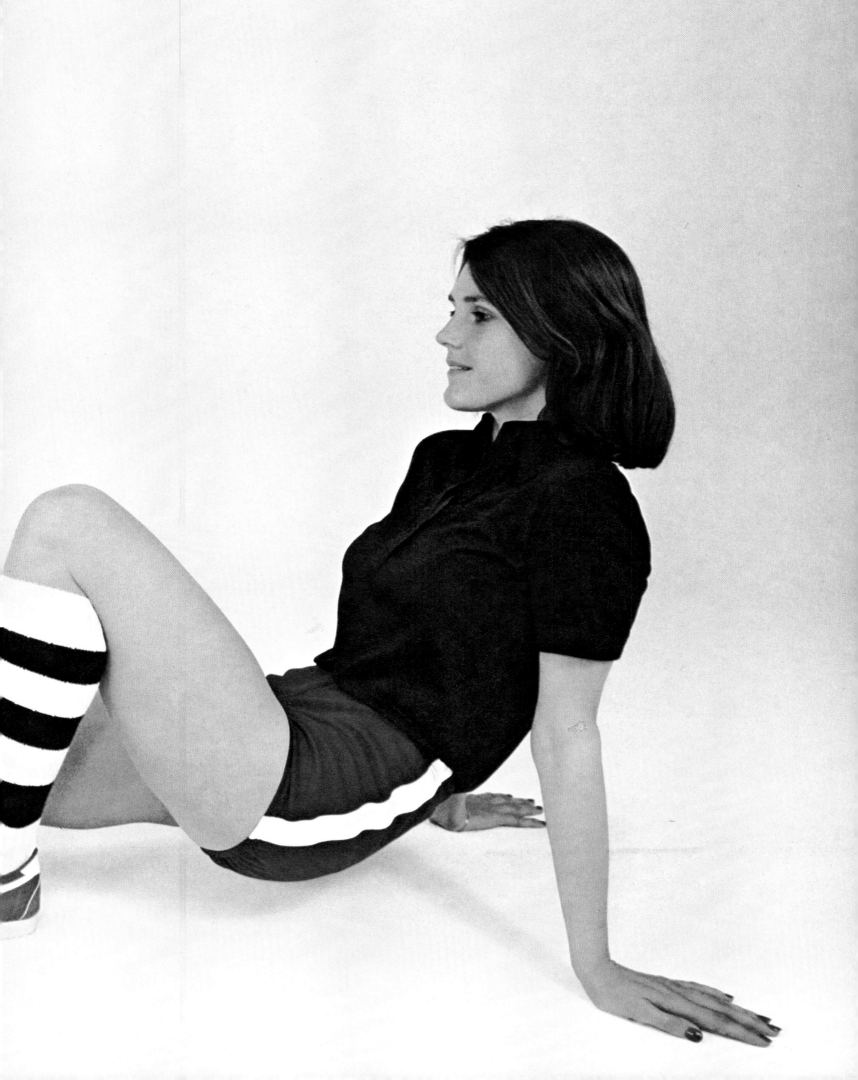

42 This Movement Pattern is similar to the previous one and strengthens your arms, thighs and abdomen. Remember to continue the 'bouncing' motion throughout. Keep your upper body fairly upright to prevent strain on your neck. Raise your hips in B, D, F and H and lower them in C, E, G and I, keeping them off the floor throughout the sequence. Raise your leg as close to vertical as you can in D and H and always lower it to the floor gently. Perform the sequence for at least one minute.

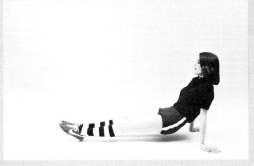

A Sit with your weight on your hands and heels, your hips off the floor, and begin to bounce lightly.

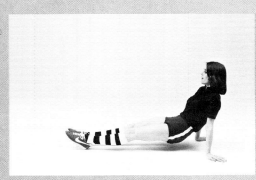

E Lower your right leg.

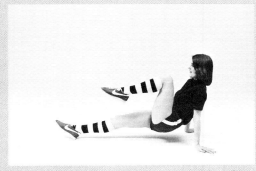

F Bring your left knee to your chest.

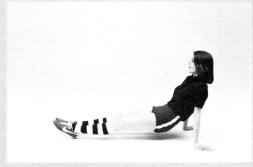

G Lower your left knee.

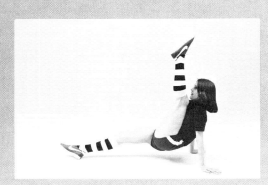

H Bring your left leg to your chest.

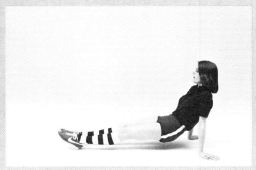

I Lower your left leg and continue, beginning with **B**.

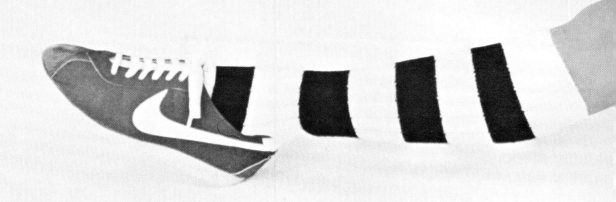

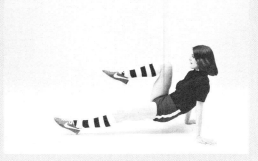

B Bring your right knee to your chest.

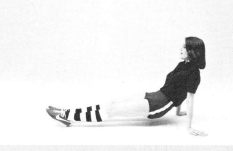

C Lower your right knee.

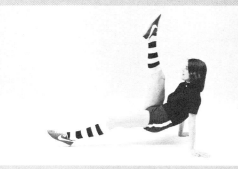

D Bring your right leg to your chest.

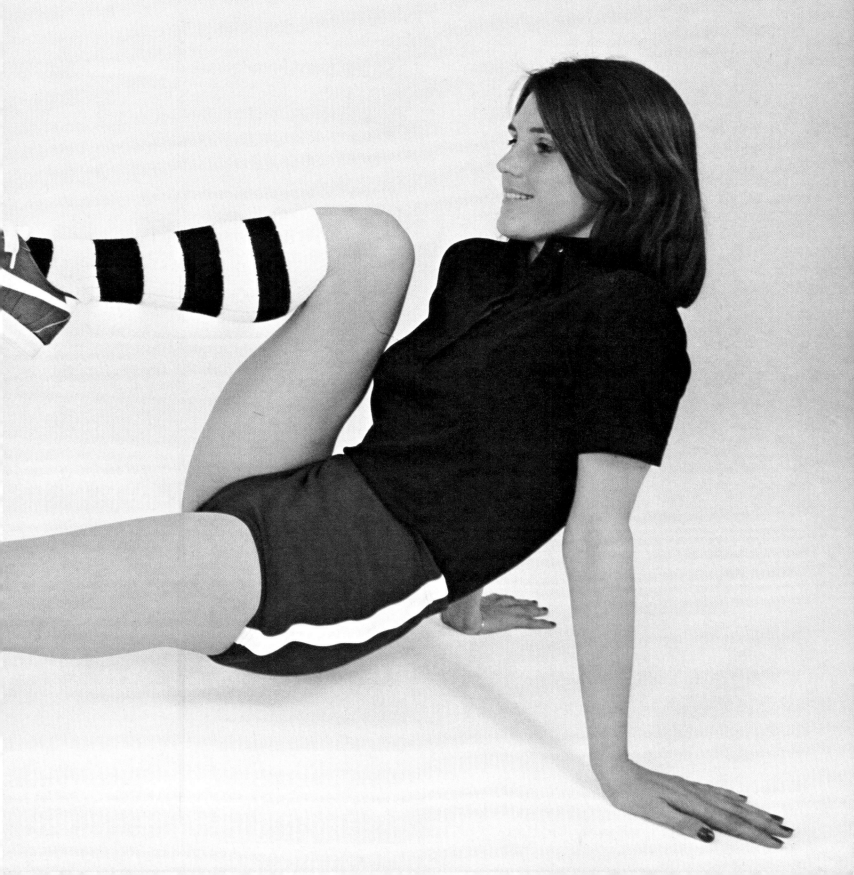

43 This Movement Pattern stretches your calf muscles and strengthens your thigh and abdominal muscles. Your lower back should be in contact with the floor throughout. Follow the movement of your foot to exercise your neck muscles.

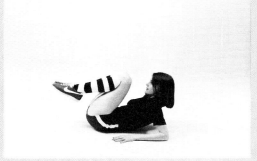

A Lie with your knees bent and your upper body slightly off the floor, supported by your elbows.

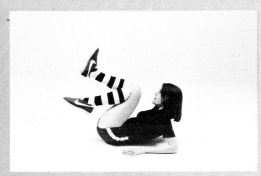

B Slowly raise your right leg.

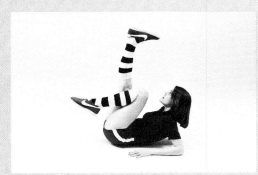

C Push your heel to the ceiling as you raise your leg.

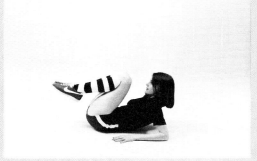

D Drop your leg and relax.

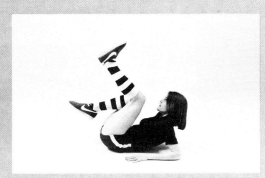

E Slowly raise your left leg.

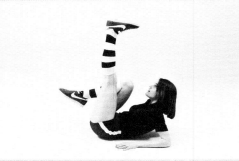

F Push your heel to the ceiling as you raise your leg.

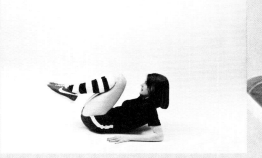

G Drop your leg and relax. Repeat, beginning with **B**.

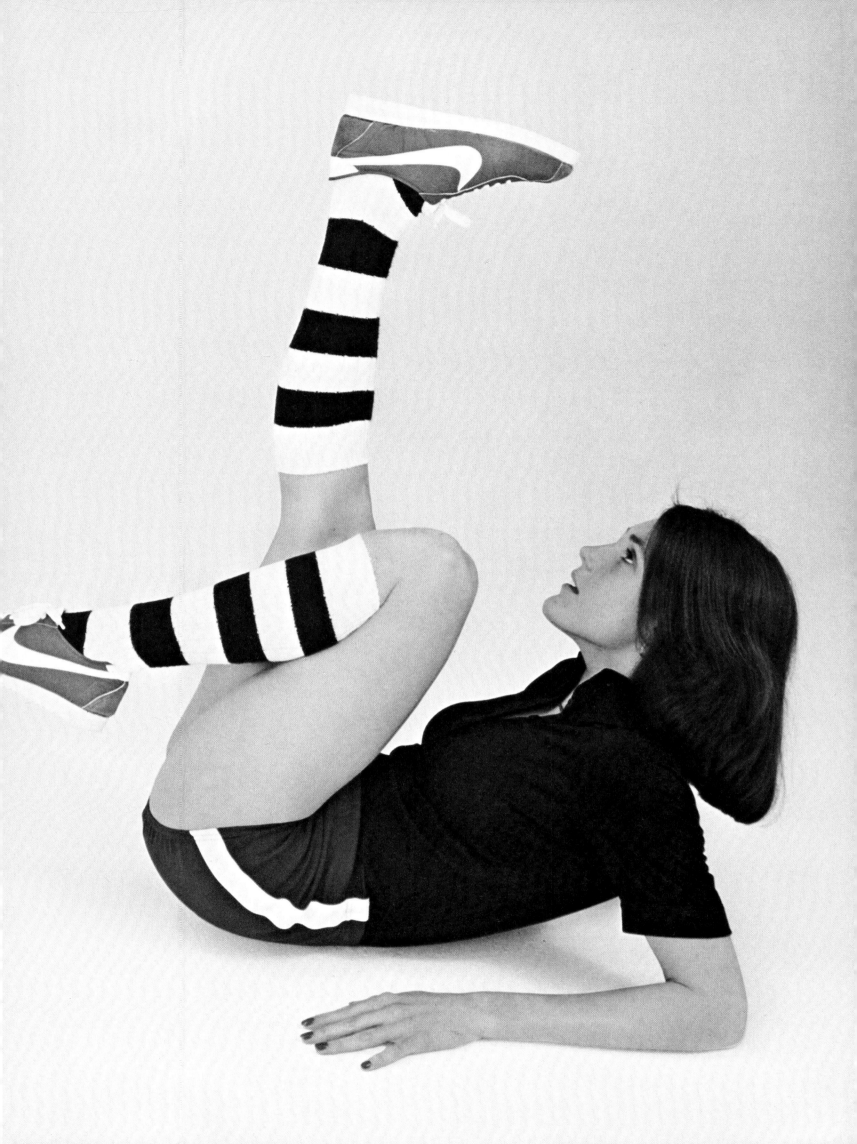

Relax

Sometimes known as the Pelvic Tilt, this deep breathing exercise renews your energy by getting more oxygen into your blood stream, strengthens your abdominal muscles and relieves tension in your lower back. Lying down also gives your muscles an opportunity to relax. Repeat this exercise until you feel rested.

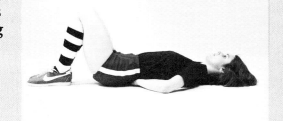

A Lie relaxed with your knees bent and your left hand beneath the small of your back, palm down.

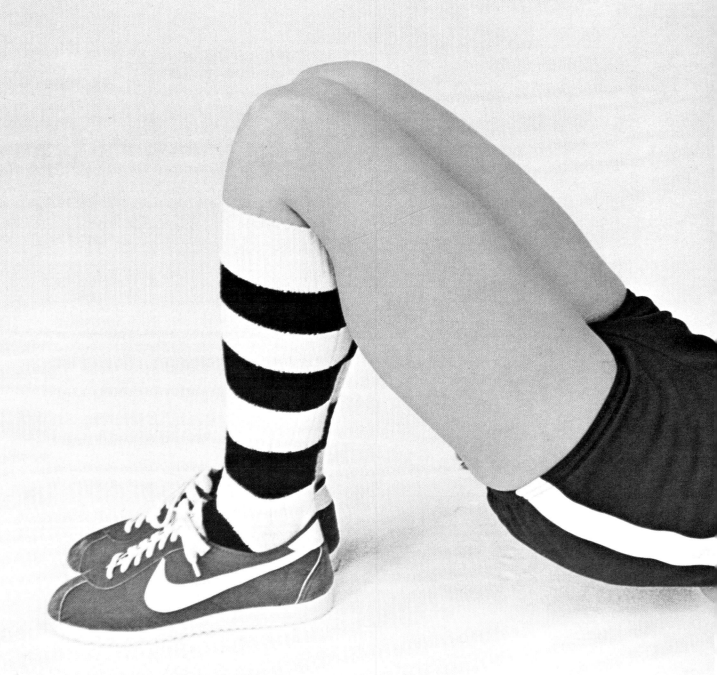

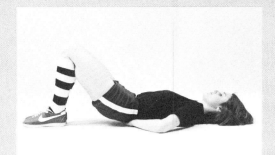 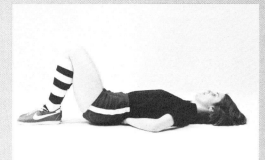

B Press your back against your hand by contracting your abdominal muscles and squeezing your buttocks together. Exhale deeply.

C Release the pressure applied in **B** and inhale deeply. Repeat the sequence, beginning with **B**.

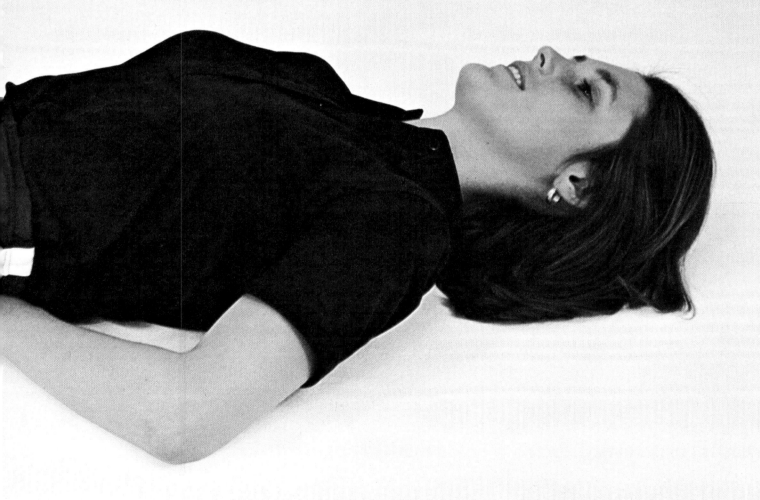

44 Each of the final Movement Patterns is performed while lying first on one side, then on the other. For convenience they are arranged so that you finish one Movement Pattern on the side on which you begin the next. These leg lifts strengthen your thighs and improve your hip flexibility. Your lower knee, bent at 90°, helps to support your back. Make sure you stay on your side throughout–not on your back. Perform each sequence briskly, from four to twelve times, first on your right side as in A, and then on your left, as in F.

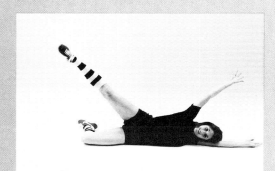

D Lower your arm and leg.

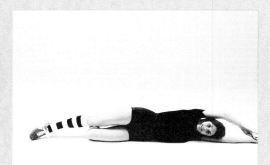

E Clap your hands overhead as your foot touches the floor then repeat, beginning with **B.**

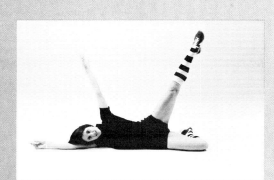

I Lower your arm and leg.

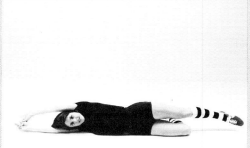

J Clap your hands overhead as your foot touches the floor then repeat, beginning with **F.**

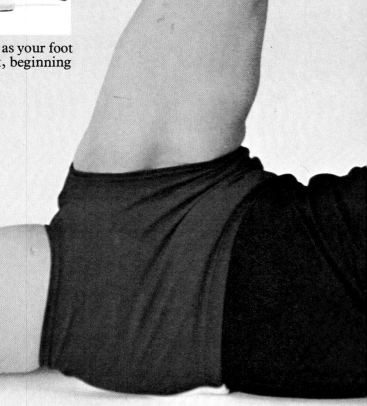

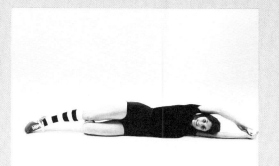

A Lie on your right side with your arms overhead and your right knee bent at 90°.

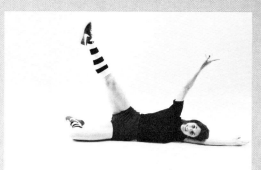

B Raise your left leg and left arm simultaneously.

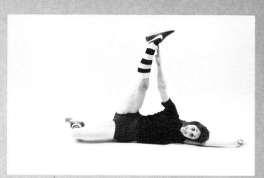

C Touch your hand to your foot.

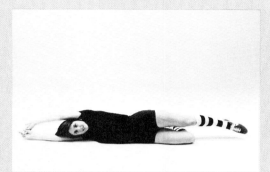

F Lie on your left side with your arms overhead and your left knee bent at 90°.

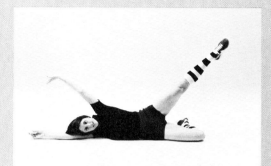

G Raise your right arm and right leg simultaneously.

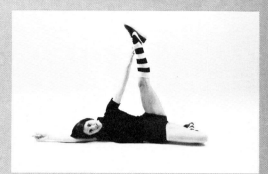

H Touch your hand to your foot.

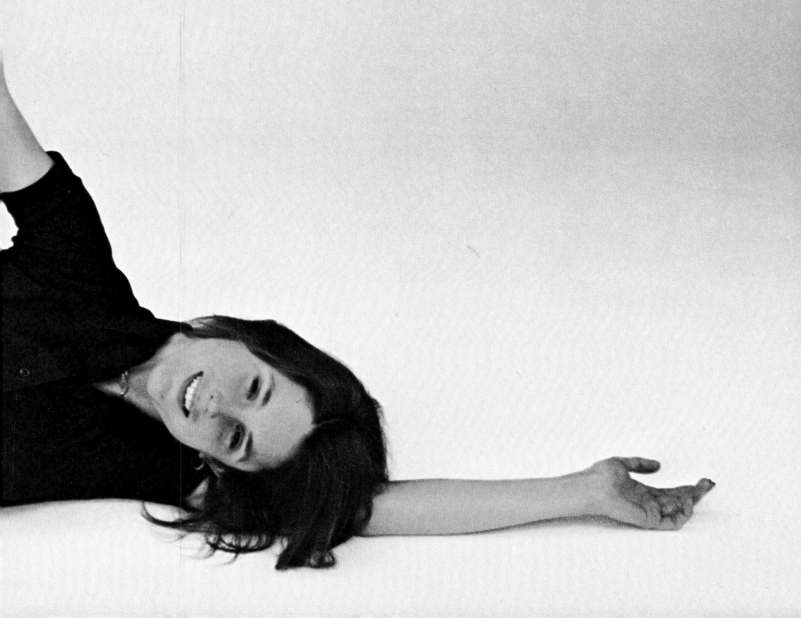

45 This Movement Pattern improves your hip flexibility and strengthens the muscles on the tops and sides of your thighs. Stay on your side throughout and make sure your lower knee is bent at 90°. Gently twist your whole leg from the hip in each case, keeping your knee locked. Keep the rest of your body still when twisting. Repeat the sequence A to F from four to twelve times then repeat G to L four to twelve times.

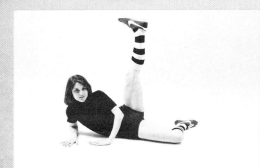

D Raise your right leg and twist it toward you. Your toe points to your head.

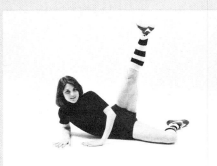

E Twist your leg away from you. Your toe points away from your head.

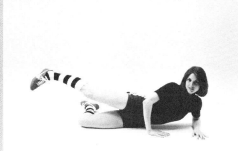

I Twist your leg to turn your toes down.

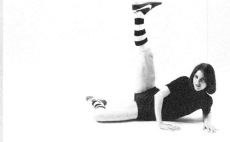

J Raise your left leg and twist it toward you. Your toe points to your head.

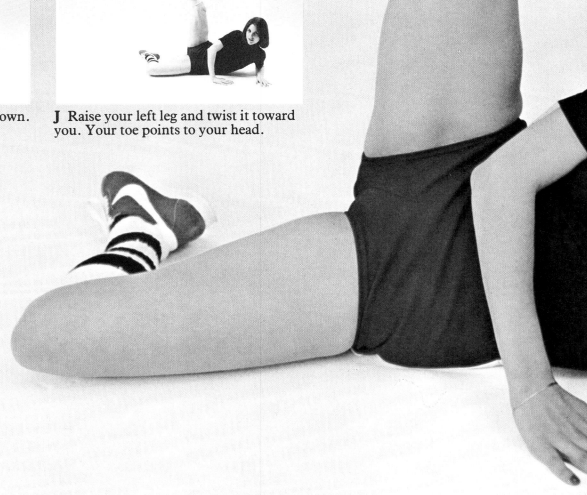

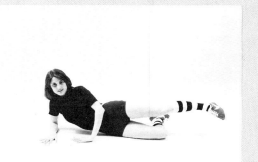 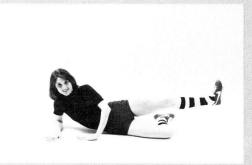 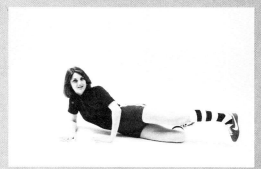

A Lie on your left side with your upper body weight on your left arm and your left knee bent at 90°.

B Extend your right leg horizontally keeping your foot flat, and twist your leg to turn your toes up.

C Twist your leg to turn your toes down.

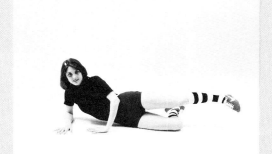 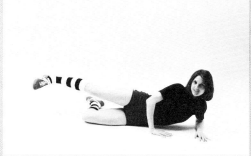 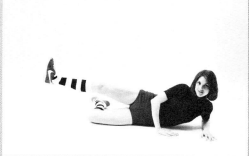

F Lower your leg and repeat, beginning with **B**.

G Lie on your right side with your upper body weight on your right arm and your right knee bent at 90°.

H Extend your left foot horizontally keeping your foot flat, and twist your leg to turn your toes up.

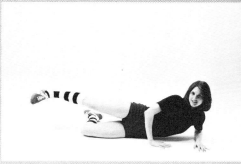

K Twist your leg away from you. Your toe points away from your head.

L Lower your leg and repeat, beginning with **H**.

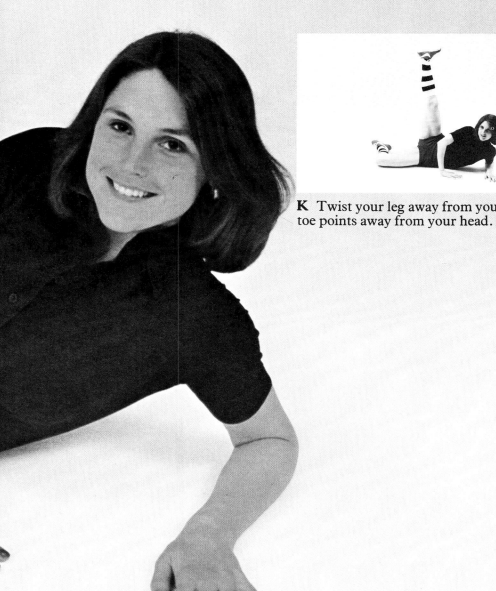

46 Flexing your knee to your shoulders stretches the inside of your thighs and improves your hip flexibility. Remember to keep your lower knee bent at 90° throughout. Perform this Movement Pattern from four to twelve times on each side.

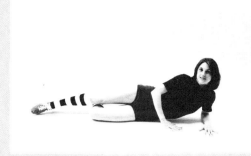

A Lie on your right side with your upper body weight on your right arm and your right knee bent at 90°.

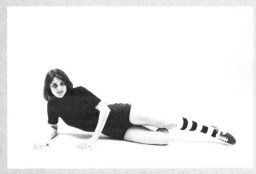

D Lie on your left side with your upper body weight on your left arm and your left knee bent at 90°.

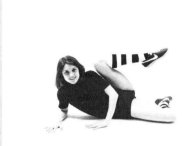

E Bend your right knee and pull it up to touch your shoulder.

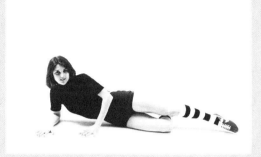

F Return your leg to the floor. Repeat **E** and **F** briskly, from four to twelve times.

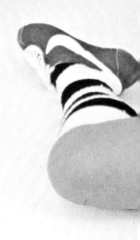

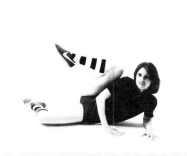 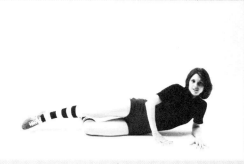

B Bend your left knee and pull it up to touch your shoulder.

C Return your leg to the floor. Repeat **B** and **C** briskly, from four to twelve times.

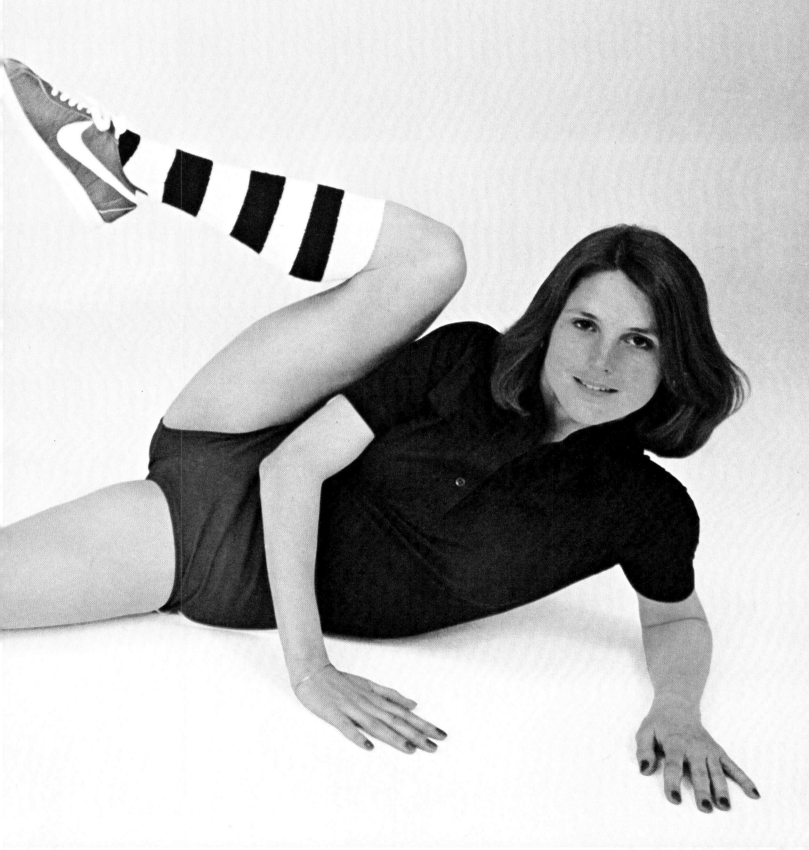

47 These hip circles improve the flexibility of your hips by taking them through a full range of movement. They are performed by describing a wide circle with your straight leg, pivoting from your hip joint. In E and K avoid reaching too far behind. Circle each leg from four to twelve times.

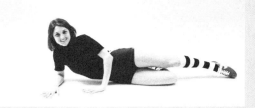

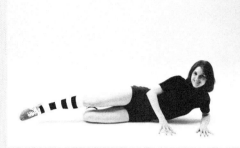

A Lie on your left side with your upper body weight on your left arm and your left knee bent at 90°.

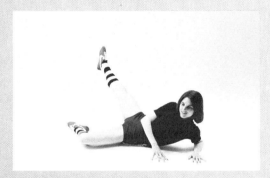

E Stop the circle above your left foot.

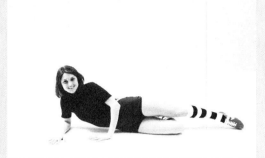

F Resume position **A** then circle forward again, beginning with **B**.

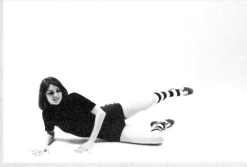

G Lie on your right side with your upper body weight on your right arm and your right knee bent at 90°.

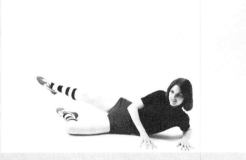

J Continue to circle back and down.

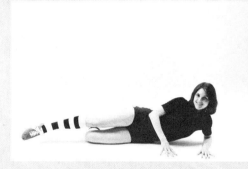

K Stop the circle above your right foot.

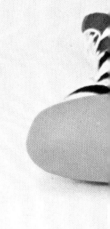

L Resume position **G** then circle forward again, beginning with **H** .

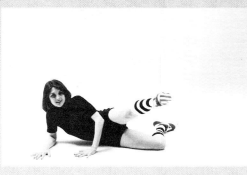

B Lock your right knee and begin a forward circle with your right leg.

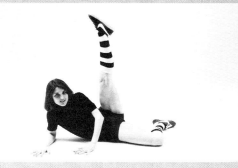

C Continue the circle high overhead.

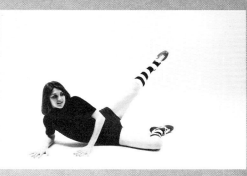

D Continue to circle back and down.

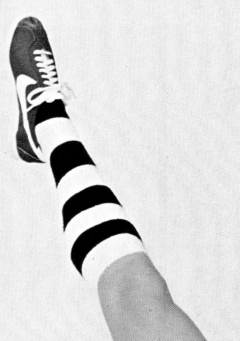

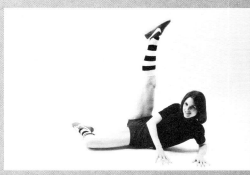

H Lock your left knee and begin a forward circle with your left leg.

I Continue the circle high overhead.

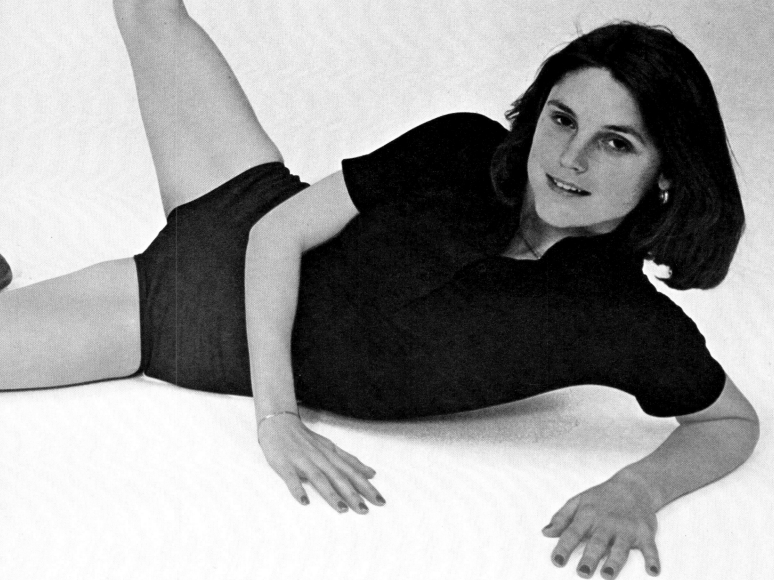

48

The final Movement Pattern strengthens your arm and torso muscles and gives your body an overall stretch. Hold positions C and H for a few seconds. Perform the sequence from four to twelve times on each side.

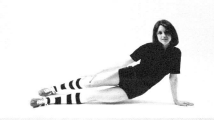

A Rest on your right side with your weight on your right hand and your left foot slightly behind your right foot.

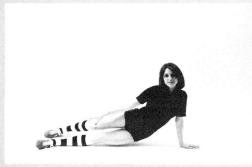

E Finish as in **A** then repeat, beginning with **B**.

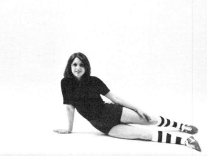

F Rest on your left side with your weight on your left hand and your right foot slightly behind your left foot.

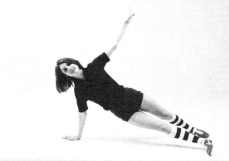

G Raise yourself on your left hand, bringing your right hand overhead.

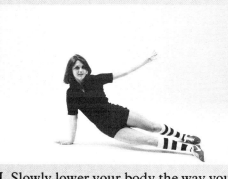

I Slowly lower your body the way you came.

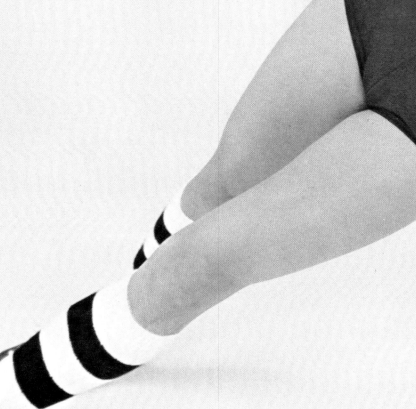

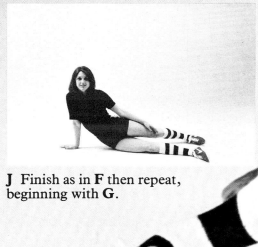

J Finish as in **F** then repeat, beginning with **G**.

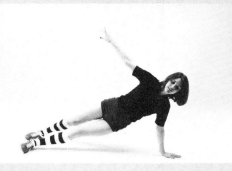

B Raise yourself on your right hand, bringing your left hand overhead.

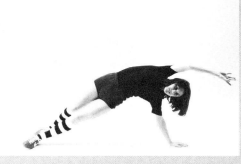

C Finish with your body raised in an arc at arm's length and your left hand extended. Hold for a few seconds.

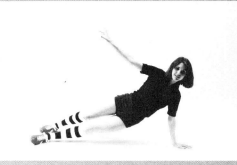

D Slowly lower your body the way you came.

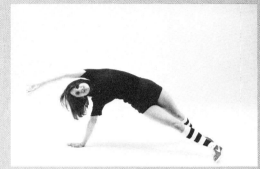

H Finish with your body raised in an arc at arm's length and your right hand extended. Hold for a few seconds.

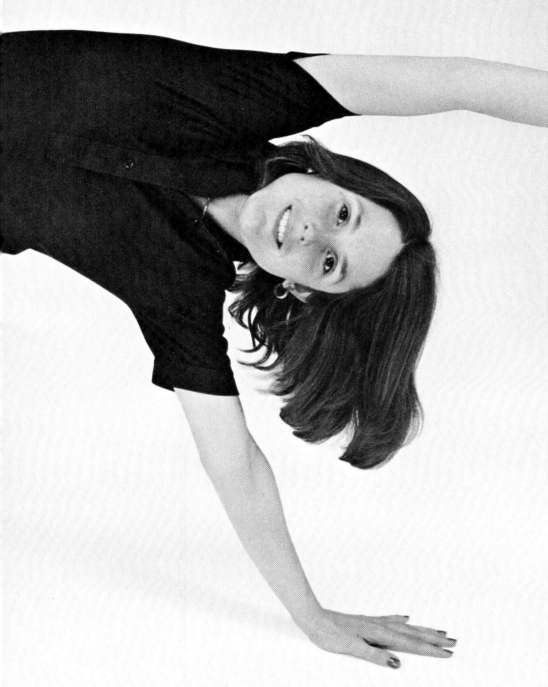

Relax

This last exercise stretches your inner thighs, but its main purpose is to renew your strength and energy and relax your body. In B reach forward only as far as comfortable then stop, keeping your back as flat as possible. In C you should be completely relaxed. Exhale as you go down in B and C. Inhale as you come up in D and E. Repeat the exercise until you feel rested.

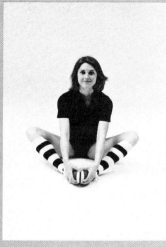

A Sit relaxed with your feet together and grasp them as shown.

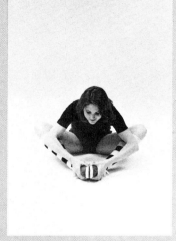

B Gently pull yourself this far toward your toes then stop, exhaling as you go.

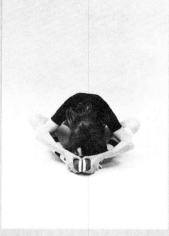

C Slump forward with your forehead on your toes and all your breath expelled.

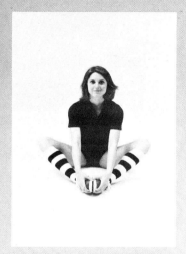

D Slowly uncurl, inhaling deeply.

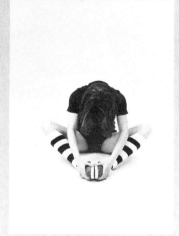

E Finish like this then repeat, beginning with **B**.

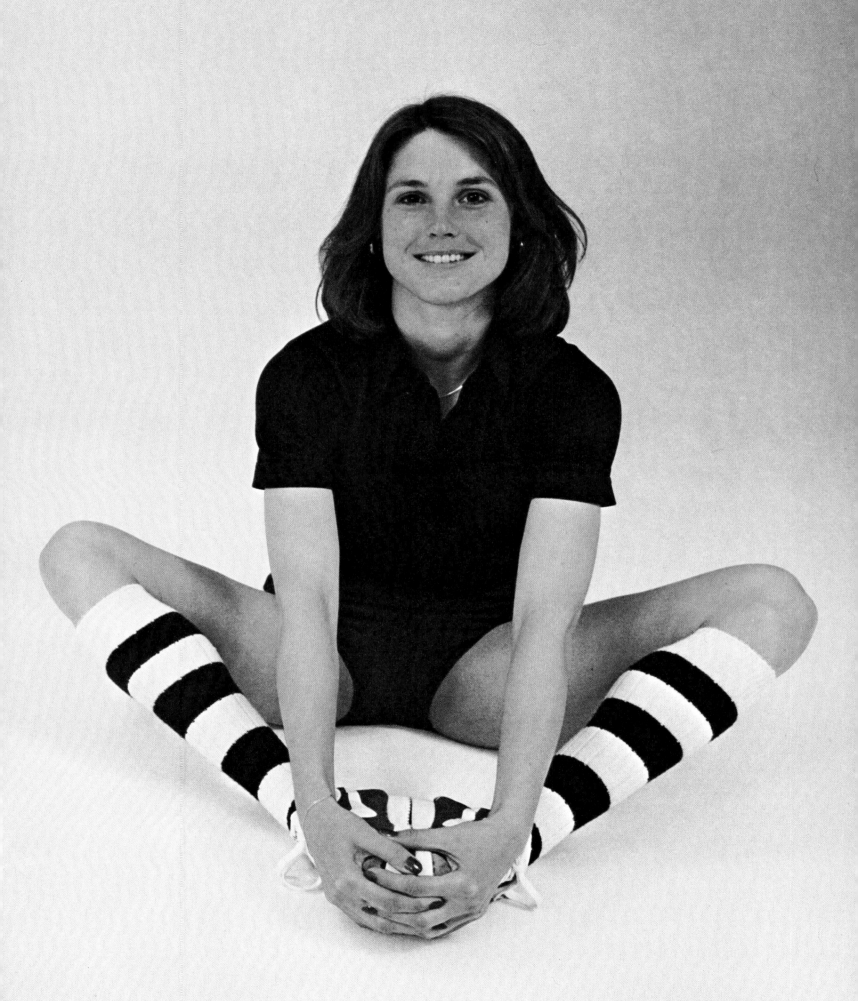

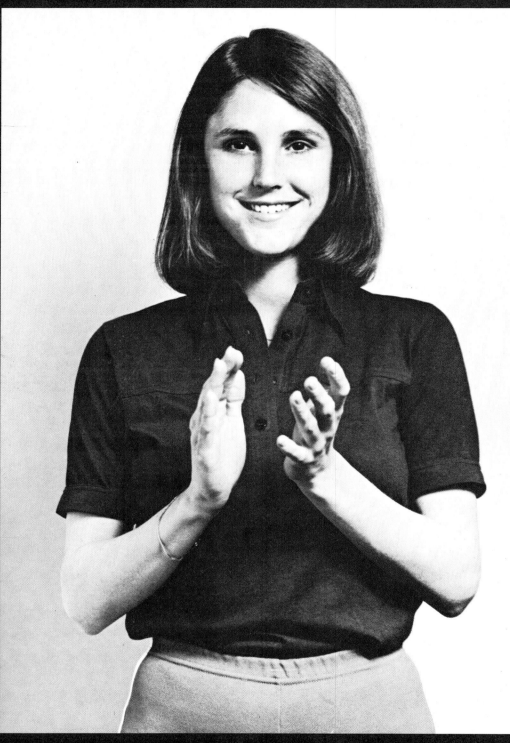

Well done!